D1806962

Experiences with primary health care in Zambia

Edited by

Joseph M. Kasonde

&

John D. Martin

World Health Organization
Geneva, Switzerland

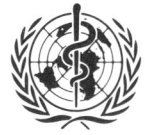

World Health Organization
Geneva
1994

WHO Library Cataloguing in Publication Data

Experiences with primary health care in Zambia / edited by Joseph M. Kasonde & John D.
 Martin.

 (Public health in action 2)

 1. Primary health care 2. National health programmes
 3. Health policy 4. Zambia I. Kasonde, Joseph M. II. Martin, John D. III. Series

 ISBN 92 4 156169 6   (NLM Classification: W 84.6)
 ISSN 1020-1629

TYPESET IN INDIA
PRINTED IN ENGLAND
93/9810-Macmillan/Clays/TWC-7500

Contents

Preface

The International Conference on Primary Health Care held in Alma-Ata in 1978 was a landmark in the history of international health. Never before or since has the commitment of the world community to health development and equity in health been so clearly articulated. But the transformation of intentions to practice had to be left to individual countries which alone could translate the Declaration of Alma-Ata into better health for their peoples. The assessment of progress and impact must therefore be based on the experiences of individual countries or communities.

This book describes the experience of one country in trying to implement primary health care. That country is Zambia, which was officially designated as a least developed country in 1991 after two decades of serious economic decline.

WHO is publishing this book as part of its efforts to stimulate more thought, discussion and action on the complex issue of how to make primary health care work. In choosing Zambia, WHO is demonstrating its concern to see much greater global interest and support for countries and peoples in greatest need.

The contributors to the book have all had personal involvement in implementation of the primary health care approach in Zambia at various times since the Alma-Ata Conference. Whether based in the Ministry of Health at national level, in the University of Zambia or working in district projects supported by nongovernmental organizations, their respective experiences and insights combine to provide a unique account of the complex process of establishing a health system based on primary health care.

Much time has been devoted to international debate on whether primary health care has been a success or a failure. It seems to us that this is a futile exercise which reflects a serious lack of understanding of the fact that health development will always depend on a number of fundamental factors, and particularly on economic development. The principles of primary health care are guidelines whose application will increase a country's ability to achieve health for all, but only within the parameters of its own economic realities. Thus, in the case of Zambia, the spiralling decline which set in during the early 1970s has been a major obstacle.

Nevertheless, WHO remains convinced that the principles of primary health care, beginning with equity, are the only means of achieving a meaningful improvement in the health of entire populations. The challenge of how to bring this to operational reality has turned out to be much more complex, difficult and exacting than had been foreseen.[1]

The fact that primary health care can work is evidenced by many examples, both small and large in scale, from around the world. Zambia provides some such examples. Nevertheless, it is as yet rare to find entire national systems that are able to sustain the primary health care approach successfully.

What are the ingredients of success? The WHO Consultative Committee on Primary Health Care Development identified the following criteria.[1] We reproduce them to assist the reader in analysing the Zambian experience:

— persisting national political, social and financial commitment, with clear policy and administrative guidelines that reach to the periphery;

— strong management capabilities that can implement the programmes, including management information systems that track equity and effectiveness and point towards those who are especially at risk;

— health personnel oriented and trained so as to understand and have their own commitment to the implementation of primary health care;

— decentralization to district and subdistrict levels so that management decisions can be made with close relevance to local conditions;

— community participation with active involvement in local decisions about primary health care planning and implementation;

— sustained financing, preferably with community input to the extent that it will engender a sense of ownership but without inhibition of usage;

— primary health care programmes that bring life-saving technologies to individual families at costs that are affordable even in the midst of poverty.

It remains to be seen whether or not the experiences described in this volume constitute success. But they certainly confirm our view that a prerequisite for progress in implementing primary health care programmes is the recording and analysis of previous experiences. If the chapters that follow have raised questions about the value of selected approaches to

---

[1] *Primary health care towards the year 2000: a report of the Consultative Committee on Primary Health Care Development, Geneva, 9-12 April, 1990* (unpublished document WHO/SHS/90.1, available on request from Division of Strengthening of Health Services, World Health Organization, 1211 Geneva 27, Switzerland).

primary health care and suggested answers, then the book, at least, has succeeded.

J.M. Kasonde
J.D. Martin

The editors of this book are grateful to Miss Peggy Chibuye of the University of Zambia School of Medicine, Department of Nursing, who first proposed the writing of these chapters.

CHAPTER 1

Zambia — a country profile

J.D. Martin

Zambia covers an area of 752 610 km² in central-southern Africa. It is land-locked and shares common borders with Zaire and the United Republic of Tanzania in the north, Malawi in the east, Mozambique, Zimbabwe and Namibia to the south, and Angola to the west.

Despite its large size the population is only 8 million (1990) of which 55% live in urban areas and 45% in rural areas. This population break-down makes Zambia the most urbanized country in Africa. In the rural areas the population is widely scattered with an overall population density of seven per km², although in some places such as the North Western Province this may be as low as three per km². These crude statistics illustrate both the results of a long-standing industrial orientation, with people migrating to the mining towns of the Copperbelt in search of employment, and the development challenges of the post-1970s during which time the Zambian economy has suffered one of the world's steepest and most sudden downturns. In 1991 Zambia was one of six countries which dropped from the middle-income category to that of least developed. How can Zambia cope with the unemployed, the underemployed and growing poverty in the cities and towns? How can Zambia provide financial, technical and social support to the scattered small farmers so as to develop the neglected rural economy? How can Zambia sustain a system of health care which can deliver effective curative and preventive services to the majority of the population, sufficient to halt and then reverse the decline in health status? These are questions that have confronted govern-ment since the economic decline began in 1975. They form the backdrop against which the story of primary health care is traced.

Legacies of pre-independence Northern Rhodesia

The Republic of Zambia came into existence on 24 October 1964, emerg-ing from the former British colony of Northern Rhodesia to become an independent state. The economy of Northern Rhodesia was built on the exploitation of the wealth of mineral deposits, mainly copper. The copper mines attracted immigrants of European descent from Southern Rhodesia (now Zimbabwe) and South Africa. They were accompanied by a small number of farmers who established often large, so-called commercial farms along the principal railway line leading south. The development of the mines also attracted large numbers of indigenous workers in search of employment, triggering the drift from rural areas and causing gradual growth of the urban population.

As in southern Africa as a whole, the European minority sought to consolidate its hold on economic and political power. In 1953 this found expression through the establishment of the Central African Federation comprising Northern Rhodesia (Zambia), Southern Rhodesia (now Zimbabwe) and Nyasaland (now Malawi), all with sizeable European settler populations. Neglect of education facilities for indigenous people and restrictions on employment opportunities were two means by which settler supremacy was to be secured. The limited expenditure on education was mainly restricted to primary schools. As a consequence, by 1960, there were only 2500 black secondary school students in the whole of Northern Rhodesia. By the time independence was attained in 1964 the country had only some 1000 persons with secondary school certificates and fewer than 100 university graduates. By contrast, Uganda had already reached this stage by 1955 and Ghana by 1943. This particular legacy has been a principal constraint to post-independence economic and social development efforts.

Health and health care in Zambia

Zambia's colonial history has had an important impact on post-independence development of the health system. Development of infrastructure had been geared towards exploitation of the copper reserves which are concentrated in one area of the country and limited resources were invested in social and economic development of the country as a whole. Such health care as existed in rural areas was provided by mission hospitals.

Against this background post-independence governments have shown impressive commitment to financing the health sector. The policy of successive governments was the provision of free health services for the entire population. Annual budgetary allocations averaged 8% of total government recurrent expenditure up to 1982. However, persistent high inflation exacted a heavy toll, resulting in a decline in real health expenditure by some 41% between 1970 and 1984. The growing pace of decline in subsequent years also led to a reduction in the health sector's share of government expenditure. The combined effect of the two trends has been dramatic. During the period 1982–1987, real per capita expenditure declined by nearly 50%, standing at US$ 2.75 in 1989.

Nevertheless, there were considerable achievements in the provision of health care. In the 20-year period from independence to 1984 the number of hospitals rose from 48 to 83, an increase of 41%. In terms of hospital beds Zambia had one of the highest levels of provision in sub-Saharan Africa. The number of health centres increased from 306 to 845 during the same period, a rise of 64%. This commitment to health care, particularly to correcting the imbalances between urban and rural areas, was paralleled in

2

other social sectors such as education. The impact on health status of these early attempts at social development was evidenced by a continuing decline in the infant mortality rate (IMR) from 147 per 1000 live births in 1969 to around 100 per 1000 in 1980. These figures disguise considerable variations within the country. In general, the IMR has been higher in rural areas. Unfortunately, there is evidence that these achievements have been undermined in recent years. This trend has been linked to effects of the deteriorating economy such as chronic undernutrition, as well as the impact of acquired immunodeficiency syndrome (AIDS). A 1992 demographic and health survey estimated that the IMR had increased to 107 deaths per 1000 live births.

In this environment of serious economic decline it has not been possible to maintain the early commitment to creating health infrastructure. The imbalance in coverage in favour of the urban population and those living along the rail link has persisted. Moreover, the pattern of allocation of government budgets has consistently favoured the large urban hospitals. In 1980, for example, it was estimated that Lusaka and the urban Copperbelt, with only 3% of the population, accounted for around 60% of national health expenditure. A 1978 analysis estimated government expenditure in urban areas at 9 kwacha per person compared with 5.50 kwacha in rural areas. This pattern was maintained as economic decline set in. Consequently it was estimated in 1984 that the health system was accessible to only 75% of the total population, accessibility being measured in terms of the numbers of people living within 12 km of a health facility. The disaggregated figure for the rural population is 50%. However, access to effective health care may in fact be considerably lower as a result of erratic and limited supplies of essential drugs and vaccines as well as of basic supplies and equipment. A 1984 evaluation found that 75% of the health centres visited had not had sufficient antimalarial drugs during the previous year. Another common problem was lack of paraffin to keep refrigerators functioning and consequent inability to support vaccination programmes, which are an essential element of primary health care. It has been argued that such basic problems illustrate the lack of priority accorded to preventive health services in comparison with hospital-based curative care. In 1984 only some 37% of infants were fully vaccinated. Fortunately the problems of the immunization programme have subsequently been successfully tackled.

The economic crisis also resulted in serious shortages of health personnel and poor morale due to low salaries seriously eroded by inflation and to deteriorating working and living conditions. The capital budget was the first to be curtailed, resulting in cutbacks in maintenance of hospitals, health centres and the already modest staff accommodation. Even when external aid was provided to support construction and maintenance, problems of lack of transport and rising costs of building materials led to very slow execution of projects. Efforts by the Ministry of Health to alleviate the problem of low morale by offering extra allowances for staff working in rural areas were thwarted by the need for government to provide similar payments to employees of all sectors, which it could not afford to do. Consequently, for example, the number of doctors in the country gradually declined. A 1987 study found that 60% of established posts were vacant. Moreover, only 13% of posts were filled by Zambian nationals. Most were filled by expatriates recruited on special contracts which included lump sum payments in foreign exchange as incentives to retain their services, although such incentives were not available to Zambian nationals.

In summary, the main factors contributing to the structure of the health system and the health status of the population were the historical background of curative orientation, lack of trained personnel and, above all, a dramatic decline in the economy as of the mid-1970s. It is against this background that the development of primary health care should be examined.

The health system

Health care in Zambia is provided by government institutions, religious missions, industries (particularly the mines), a number of parastatal companies, private practitioners, traditional healers and the armed services. Of these, the government has been the principal provider of care through a wide network of health centres and hospitals, followed by the religious missions which provide approximately 30% of total hospital beds, mainly in district and general hospitals.

During the 1980s the number of hospitals remained constant at 83. The number of health centres continued to increase steadily, following a 100% increase in the decade after independence was attained, thereby reflecting the policy of increasing the rural population's access to basic health services.

The 83 hospitals comprise three central (or tertiary) hospitals, three specialist hospitals (paediatric, psychiatric and leprosy), nine provincial hospitals located in each provincial capital and 68 district hospitals. Although the number of hospitals remained constant, the number of beds doubled, from 10 800 in 1964 to 22 800 in 1987.

Health centres provide services mainly to the rural population. Large health centres have beds for general inpatient care as well as for maternity care. Even small sub-centres may have a few beds, depending on the size of the population covered and the closeness of hospitals for referral. Health centres are staffed by paramedical personnel—medical assistants, nurses and health assistants dealing with public health services in the catchment area.

During the period up to the advent of multiparty democracy in 1991, responsibility for administration of the health care system resided with the three levels of the Ministry of Health, i.e. the central Ministry headquarters in Lusaka, nine provincial offices and 57 district offices which reported to their immediate supervisor, the Provincial Medical Officer.

The central Ministry headquarters had responsibility for formulating health policy, planning, issuing policy guidelines to the lower levels, managing national preventive health programmes such as immunization and maternal health care, and allocating funds. Approval of national health policy was the responsibility of the Central Committee of the ruling party.

Management of the implementation of primary health care nationwide was the responsibility of one of three Assistant Directors of Medical Services. The so-called essential elements of primary health care—such as maternal and child health, immunization, nutrition and health education—came within the terms of reference of this officer. These were the traditional areas of responsibility of the Ministry of Health's department of preventive services. The introduction of primary health care in 1980 brought the role of the district into focus. It was at the level of the district that the concept of primary health care became tangible. Indeed, the district was defined as the basic unit of implementation for primary health care. Each of its health units—sub-centre, health centre and district hospital—had complementary roles to play, including interaction with local communities and their traditional birth attendants, traditional healers and community health workers.

The health of the Zambian people

A remarkable demographic feature of the population of Zambia is its growth rate, which at 3.2% per year (1993) is one of the highest in the world. This reflects the long-standing low priority accorded to family planning.

Life expectancy at birth has improved considerably since independence was attained, rising from an estimated 45 years for women and 41.8 years for men to 57.5 years and 55.4 years respectively in 1992. By far the greatest toll of mortality occurs among children. However, the IMR, which is considered a rough but useful indicator of social development, fell considerably in the period up to 1980. Accurate figures are difficult to obtain since so many births take place at home. Nevertheless, available statistics indicate a rate of 147 deaths per 1000 live births for 1969 which declined to around 100 per 1000 in the period 1980–1985. These are national averages which conceal higher levels of mortality in rural areas, especially in Luapula and Northern Provinces. Even in urban areas considerable variations occur, with very poor squatter compounds registering three times the rate of low density middle-class areas.

Communicable diseases are the major causes of mortality and morbidity in Zambia. They include malaria, diarrhoea, acute respiratory infections, measles, meningitis and tuberculosis. Other common causes of mortality and morbidity are malnutrition and accidents. AIDS has become a serious public health problem since 1985, particularly in urban areas. A number of studies have shown that up to 30% of admissions to urban hospitals are HIV-related. Serious outbreaks of cholera have occurred each year since 1989, particularly affecting Northern, Luapula and Copperbelt Provinces.

Malaria is endemic and is one of the top three causes of mortality and morbidity in all age groups. There was an increase in the numbers of cases and deaths during the 1980s, resulting from resistance to treatment by chloroquine and other antimalarials as well as ineffective control measures.

Admissions to hospitals for tuberculosis have more than doubled since 1984 and may be related to HIV infection. The number of cases recorded in 1990 was 16 838 compared with 6747 in 1985. This rise has been accompanied by an increase in the case-fatality rate.

Malnutrition has been a persistent problem in Zambia and is a major cause of death in the 1–14-year age group. A study by the University Teaching Hospital in Lusaka reported that malnutrition, as a cause of death in those aged 1 to 14, rose from 18.5% in 1974 to 62.2% in 1984. A 1992 study reports that 50% of three-year-olds are stunted—that is, below the normal height for their age. This reflects chronic undernutrition. The problem is more serious in rural areas, particularly in Northern and Luapula provinces. The incidence of malnutrition increases during the pre-harvest season, from November to March, when food stocks have been depleted. Not surprisingly, this has come to be known as the "hungry season".

The introduction of the primary health care approach in 1980 was intended to respond to this array of serious but preventable health problems and to bring about a shift of emphasis from curative care to prevention and health promotion. In this respect immunization has been a notable success. Between 1983 and 1990 the proportions of fully immunized children rose from 37% to 73%. Another indicator of progress has been the proportion of pregnant women receiving antenatal care—up from 60% to 80% in the same period. This is offset by the fact that only one-third of babies are delivered with the assistance of medically trained personnel.

The chapters that follow trace the history of implementation of primary health care in Zambia. The reader may find it useful to refer back to this brief account of the health status of the Zambian people and the development of the health system which preceded primary health care. No country can start from scratch. Primary health care must take account of the past as well as the prevailing economic realities.

CHAPTER 2

Moving towards primary health care [1]

J.M. Kasonde & J.D. Martin

The development of a health care system containing elements of primary health care was already under way in Zambia before 1978. The Alma-Ata Conference gave considerable impetus and direction to this process and, as a consequence, the Government of Zambia decided to adopt primary health care as the main focus in further development of its national health services.

The planning process

Existing policies already called for free medical services for all the people of Zambia, and the five-year development plan emphasized the need to give priority to the rural population, whose needs were greatest. Community participation through self-help projects is a long-established tradition in Zambia, as evidenced by the fact that some 30% of existing rural health centres were built on a self-help basis.

These factors favoured the introduction of primary health care, despite a considerable bias towards the urban population, in the form of large sophisticated hospitals, and towards highly cure-oriented health services in the country as a whole.

From the outset the Ministry of Health fully realized the importance of intersectoral cooperation in planning and implementing primary health care. As a first step, a National Coordinating Committee was established, drawing its membership from the United National Independence Party, relevant government ministries (Agriculture and Water Development, Education, Information and Broadcasting, Finance, and Community Development) and the churches' medical association.

This well-intentioned experiment in intersectoral cooperation was to prove the first of many problems that would be encountered. The committee failed to function because the participants from the non-health sectors felt unable to contribute in the absence of specific proposals from the Ministry of Health. As a result, the Ministry of Health decided to produce its own detailed proposals for the introduction of primary health care, which would be presented to the National Coordinating Committee for

---

[1] This chapter first appeared in *World health forum*, 1983, 4: 25–30.

approval and thereafter would be submitted for nationwide discussion by all involved sectors and by the general public.

It was realized that this "top–down" approach would be criticized as contrary to the community initiative advocated by most proponents of primary health care. Yet it was concluded that the most practical way of achieving a workable primary health care system was to present proposals dealing with all aspects of organization so that people could appreciate how their needs and expectations fitted into the overall national framework and, particularly, so that they could appreciate the extent of available resources and modify their expectations to a realistic level. In addition, it was strongly felt that productive discussion required the presence of people who were aware of the overall national circumstances and who could appropriately and directly respond to questions and comments.

Two bodies were established for the purpose of preparing proposals. The first was a Primary Health Care Planning Committee, which included all heads of departments within the Ministry of Health and the country representatives of the World Health Organization (WHO) and the United Nations Children's Fund (UNICEF). This committee was served by the second body, a full-time planning unit headed by an assistant director of medical services and comprising a specialist in community health, a health architect and a health planner.

The planning committee quickly identified the major problems to be tackled, which, essentially, presented a strong case in favour of a major reallocation of resources towards the rural areas and towards prevention of disease. The committee also suggested a practical administrative structure for implementing and sustaining primary health care activities at the community level. The task was completed over a period of six months and was finalized by the publication of proposals for primary health care in January 1980 in a document entitled *Health by the people: proposals for achieving health for all in Zambia*.

The primary health care document

It was intended that the document on primary care would be read and discussed not just by high officials in central ministries but also by community leaders in all districts of Zambia. Considerable effort therefore went into producing a document that was clearly and simply written, contained sufficient information yet was not so long as to discourage readers, and was attractively presented in a brightly coloured cover to avoid the initial suspicion that this was just another official report. The yellow cover greatly helped efforts to publicize the document's contents and led to a more familiar title, "The yellow book", the name by which the document has become known throughout the country.

The document was divided into a number of sections, beginning with a chapter summarizing the relevance of the primary health care approach in the Zambian context and an outline of the proposals for achieving the

8

required services. This was included to inform those, such as the press and politicians, who wanted a clear grasp of the proposals without reading the entire 100 pages. The value of including this section has been amply illustrated by the direct quotations from the chapter that have appeared in many newspaper articles and political speeches.

Other sections presented a review of the health sector performance since independence, highlighting the existing focus on urban-based curative care; proposals for organizing primary health care, with emphasis on community participation and intersectoral cooperation; a number of technical chapters dealing with tasks to be undertaken by the Ministry of Health in order to strengthen the infrastructure to support primary health care (e.g. manpower development, construction and upgrading of health centres, health education, transport); and, finally, a timetable for implementation.

The consultation process

The task of publicizing the proposals for primary health care and promoting discussion began at national level and moved through provincial and district levels to the people in their communities.

Health personnel at national and provincial levels were chosen to initiate and guide discussion because they were readily available for preliminary training and had already been consulted during the preparation of the proposals. Subsequently, health workers at district level were trained, through seminars at provincial level, to fulfil the same role in the discussions in their districts.

This direct communication with and guidance by people knowledgeable about the national health situation gave considerable assurance that the discussions would be truly productive. The procedure also had the advantage of enabling these health personnel to report the results of the discussions quickly to the Ministry of Health.

The process of consultation actually started with a one-day seminar in each provincial capital during February and March 1980. Primary health care proposals were introduced by the community health specialist from the Ministry of Health's Planning Unit (the national coordinating officer for primary health care), supported by the provincial medical officer and health education officer. Participants included senior provincial and district politicians, heads of government departments, church leaders and representatives of voluntary organizations.

The proposals were very favourably received in all provinces except the Copperbelt, a highly industrial and urbanized province well provided for by a network of hospitals catering for the curative needs of the population. In this province many people feared that the emphasis on preventive and promotive activities through primary health care would divert resources from their curative services. This fear was not dispelled until experience in the implementation of primary health care in other provinces became known.

The considerable publicity given to the seminars helped to generate much public interest. This was heightened by the coverage given to a national primary health care conference in April 1980, which was attended by some 300 persons representing national, provincial and district Party and government interests, as well as traditional healers, voluntary organizations, the churches and the press. The primary health care approach was unanimously accepted at this national gathering. Some of the original proposals contained in "The yellow book" were amended, and mental health was added to the list of primary services. The national conference was followed, from May 1980 until September 1981, by seminars at district level, which were attended by more than 10 000 people.

By the end of 1980 the Ministry of Health had received sufficient feedback to publish a final document on primary health care, entitled *Health by the people: implementing primary health care in Zambia.* Modelled closely on "The yellow book", this document set out firm and detailed guidelines for implementing primary health care, emphasizing the key role of the districts and the necessity for decentralizing responsibility for primary care to district level. The document thus recognized the considerable variations among districts and their right to establish their own health priorities.

Adoption of the final document

Responsibility for formulating national policy in Zambia lay at that time with the United National Independence Party, acting through its national council and the central committee.

The final document was submitted to the Party for consideration, and primary health care was formally approved as a national programme of the Party and its government following adoption by the central committee in August 1981.

Implementation

Implementation formally began in August 1981 with the formation of community health committees and selection of community health workers (including traditional birth attendants) for training, although initiatives had already been taken in many districts.

Strengthening of the infrastructure of the health sector, particularly within the districts, had already begun as early as January 1980, following publication of "The yellow book". This process involved a number of elements:

- Primary health care coordinators were established as a special cadre of health workers at district level to spearhead development of primary health care.
- Existing health workers were trained for their new roles in primary health care.

- Rural health centres were constructed or upgraded to provide adequate coverage of facilities for preventive and curative services and for the supervision and continued training and support of community health workers and traditional birth attendants.
- There was personnel development, with emphasis on the training of new workers to staff health facilities within the districts more adequately.
- Distribution of medicines was improved to ensure that adequate supplies of essential medicines reached the district hospitals, rural health centres and community health workers. (Although primary health care is mainly preventive, the curative aspect is an essential part, and great importance is attached to it by the general public.)
- The transport system was strengthened as a prerequisite for good organization and supervision of primary health care activities in a country with a huge land area and a thinly distributed rural population.
- Planning and management were strengthened at all levels, and particularly at district level, in order to increase the effectiveness of support for primary health care activities within the health sector and to facilitate a high degree of decentralized decision-making from central to district level.

Of all these components, the strengthening of planning and management at district level was regarded as the most important since the success of the other components and the overall implementation of primary health care depend on its effectiveness. Since the resources available for health care are limited, good management is essential to ensure that what is available is used to greatest effect.

In cooperation with the Netherlands Government, through WHO and the British Council, the Ministry of Health initiated a country health programming exercise in March 1981. Activities during 1981 concentrated on the training of staff from the offices of the nine provincial medical officers and the subsequent establishment of provincial management teams. This process required four two-week workshops at central level and visits to some provinces to assess follow-up activities by the participants. An additional one-week workshop was conducted to train the health inspector and health education officer from each province so that they could in turn train the district staff, an exercise carried out during the first half of 1982.

Training material for the workshops was developed jointly by members of the Ministry of Health Planning Unit and a consultant sponsored by the British Council. At the trainers' workshop held in August 1981, the material was reviewed and agreement was reached on the main guidelines for the production of a training manual for the 1982 district workshops. Such a manual was regarded as essential to ensure the standard training of all district staff and to give detailed guidance to trainers who conducted the workshops without assistance from Ministry of Health staff. In fact, two manuals were produced, one for "learners", containing practical exercises to be carried out, with accompanying technical information, and one for "trainers", containing the same material but with additional guidelines on how to conduct each exercise and answers to questions.

The objectives of the district workshops were to teach participants to use improved working methods in district management teams (to be formed after each workshop), to prepare district health plans in cooperation with provincial staff, and to implement and monitor the health plans that were prepared. Participants included not only health workers but also administrative and finance staff.

Following formal approval of the primary health care programme, community health committees were formed in approximately 450 communities throughout Zambia. During the last three months of 1981, candidates selected by these communities were given an initial six weeks' training.

It is probable that these were already the most articulate and best organized communities rather than those most in need of help. This raises a fundamental issue about the nature of community participation in primary health care. Is it acceptable to present ideas and proposals to people and proceed to help those who come forward, irrespective of their need, or should the government first identify those in greatest need and offer assistance irrespective of their desire or ability to participate? The Zambian conclusion was that establishing primary health care services is necessarily a very long-term process that could not succeed without the enthusiastic involvement of the people at all stages. Therefore, willingness to participate was regarded as the principal criterion for offering assistance and support, in the expectation that such "pioneer communities" would act as an example and inspiration to others. Another, more pragmatic reason for adopting this approach was that the national health system, at this early stage of primary health care development, could cope with the initial demand and at the same time work to strengthen and expand the infrastructure and thus facilitate a gradual increase in demand and activity at the community level.

The task of publicizing the experiences of the "pioneer communities" was greatly assisted by the introduction of a bimonthly primary health care news bulletin, published in 6000 copies by the Ministry of Health and distributed to all health institutions, some schools, and officers of district councils throughout the country.

Problems in developing primary health care

Though undoubted progress was achieved in developing primary health care in Zambia in a relatively short time, a number of problems were encountered.

- Within the health sector itself, support for primary health care among doctors was very limited, no doubt reflecting their conventional training and their aspirations for clinical careers and a comfortable lifestyle in urban areas. This lack of support had a strong negative influence on primary health care development. Most progress was made in provinces and districts where there was enthusiastic support by medical officers.
- Among other sections of the health staff, support for primary health care was much greater. However, despite acknowledgement of the vital importance of health education, there was reluctance to accept health education as a task to be undertaken by all health workers.
- The emphasis on prevention of sickness and promotion of good health in primary health care had little genuine public appeal. Public pressure throughout the country was for health development in terms of expansion of curative services, which led to considerable pressure on community health workers to concentrate on curative activities, although there was some evidence to suggest that activities in nutrition, water supply, sanitation and family planning captured modest public interest and support.
- The proclaimed acceptance of the need to redistribute resources more fairly in favour of areas of greatest need (mainly rural) was not matched by action. The distribution of money, personnel and medicines remained proportionately the same as it had been two years earlier when the problem was first brought to public attention. To some extent this reflected the considerable urban bias that existed in national affairs, a bias reflected and reinforced by the media, whose coverage of rural affairs was minimal and whose publicity regarding urban health matters consequently led to undue political pressure on the Ministry of Health.
- The economic depression felt in Zambia as in other developing countries in Africa resulted in general reluctance to introduce new programmes.
- The financial system was highly centralized, and the undoubted difficulty of accounting for expenditure made financial managers disinclined to release funds for activities at district and community levels. This attitude was reinforced by a relative lack of awareness on the part of finance and administrative staff of the living conditions and health problems of most of the population.
- Teamwork among health personnel at all levels, from health centre to Ministry of Health headquarters was poor. This reflected their training, which until a short time previously stressed individual technical skills rather than the additional management skills that are so vital in primary health care. A further aspect of this problem was poor cooperation among different levels of the health system.
- At community level, difficulties were encountered in sustaining the activities of health committees following the selection and training of

community health workers. A 1982 survey revealed that about 50 of the 450 committees needed to be revivified. Although the precise reasons for their inactivity were not known, it is likely that at least some communities perceived the role of the community health worker to be mainly curative and thus the role of the health committees to be solely to solve problems, such as issues of payment, when they arose.

Conclusion

Zambia's early experience in promoting primary health care was encouraging, mainly as a consequence of public enthusiasm. Many anticipated problems arose, despite attempts to forestall them. Among these, the difficulty of gaining the support of trained medical personnel was the most notable. Problems such as this underline the long and uphill tasks involved in developing successful primary health care, a task not just of education, but of re-education, in which new information and attitudes must compete with, and eventually overcome, the old.

CHAPTER 3

Planning, design and implementation of primary health care

K.G. Lowther & M.M. Moonde

The Ministry of Health of Zambia agreed in 1980 to collaborate with Africare, an American nongovernmental organization (NGO), in a pilot project to show the importance of environmental sanitation and appropriate technology in promoting primary health care in Zambia.

The project was designed jointly and Africare secured funding from another American NGO, the Christian Children's Fund, in early 1982. The project began formally in September 1982 after the Ministry appointed a senior health inspector to be the resident project coordinator in two pilot districts, Luangwa and the eastern part of Lusaka Rural.

The project remained active until late 1990 but fell far short of its original goals. While wells were dug, latrines built and community health workers trained, one of the project's main results was to underscore the need for thorough pre-project consultation and consensus-building among all concerned.

Project design

Africare, an organization with substantial experience in supporting village-based primary health care elsewhere in Africa, began supporting rural development in Zambia in 1978. It established a working relationship with the Ministry of Health and took part in a national workshop in April 1980 that introduced Zambia's primary health care strategy to potential donors. Subsequently the NGO agreed to support the pilot project in Luangwa and Lusaka Rural.

The selection of Luangwa District and Lusaka Rural District seemed logical. Both districts had been neglected in the provision of health services because they were in Lusaka Province and were considered near to the large hospital and other health facilities of Lusaka. Yet people in the eastern part of Lusaka Rural and in Luangwa actually lived between 160 and 300 km from the capital's health facilities. It was a case of "so near yet so far". Consciously or otherwise, the Ministry had tended to look beyond districts which lay within the capital's shadow and concentrate on more distant regions.

The choice of project area also seemed proper in view of the virtual shutdown of health and other public services there during the latter years of the independence struggle in neighbouring Zimbabwe. The war often spilled across the Zambezi River into both districts, making development difficult and the provision of essential services dangerous. The primary health care project was seen as a means to start drawing the area back into the flow of national life.

Finally, the Ministry of Health recommended Luangwa and Lusaka Rural because they were near Lusaka, which would make monitoring and supervision easier.

Design of the project began in December 1980 when the Africare representative in Zambia and a member of the Ministry's Primary Health Care Secretariat attended a primary health care workshop for local government staff from Lusaka Province.

The Africare/Ministry of Health design team spent two weeks in early 1981 visiting villages in Luangwa and Lusaka Rural, speaking with traditional leaders, ward chairmen, health workers and others in order to find out what the area's main health-related needs were. They confirmed that water was one of the most urgent requirements. The design team saw few latrines and heard that people thought they needed so much work that they were not worth building. There was hardly any sign of community self-help projects, and a Catholic priest told the team that the people in Luangwa were resistant to new ideas.

Field notes taken during visits to about two dozen villages, and in meetings with local leaders, civil servants and party officials, reveal in hindsight that neither the villagers nor those who would have a role in implementing the project really understood or supported primary health care.

The concept of the project originated in the Ministry of Health. It was imposed, with good intentions, on two districts whose response was passive. That passivity should have alerted the planners. However, the information gathered at village level confirmed the view of the Ministry and the planners that health problems in the area were largely traceable to poor water and sanitation.

The project was designed to meet people's clearly expressed desire for cleaner and more reliable supplies of water, to improve sanitation by introducing improved, ventilated pit latrines (decidedly not an expressed need) and to expand the number of community health workers and clinic-based health professionals. The design assumed (optimistically, it turned out) that the community health workers and the extra staff at the rural health centres would carry the burden of educating people about the importance of using latrines and encouraging them to adopt other appropriate technologies for storing water and food.

The planning process allowed for review of the project document which was drafted by the Africare representative, by the Ministry of Health and by the respective district councils. The Ministry accepted the draft and the district councils gave pro forma endorsements. There was, however, no attempt to engage the councils or their executives in a comprehensive review of the project objectives nor, most importantly, in an agreement over who would be responsible for what.

Implementation, 1982–1985

The project was intended to complement the Ministry's plan to build up a team of Zambian community health workers as part of the national primary health care strategy. The money was to finance construction or restoration of 100 wells, introduction of appropriate technologies to reduce environmental factors likely to cause disease, and the construction of staff houses at the understaffed rural health centres. The construction of wells and staff houses was on a self-help basis with materials supplied by the project and labour provided by the local community.

The project was to demonstrate environmental aspects of primary health care before their wider application in the Ministry's 10-year campaign to equip people with the knowledge and means to improve their health. The basis of the project was that a clean environment is essential for good health. The plan was to place emphasis on provision of safe and adequate water supplies. Where the people showed interest, they were to be helped to construct latrines of various designs, as well as simple devices to store water and to process and preserve food.

The Ministry of Health assigned a senior health inspector to act as resident project coordinator. Health inspectors are trained in environmental sanitation and appropriate technology. The project coordinator was to work closely with community health workers, village health committees, rural health centre staff, local leaders, district councils and other government bodies.

The Assistant Director of Medical Services (Planning) was to supervise a project management team comprising the Ministry's primary health care adviser, the Lusaka primary health care coordinator and the Lusaka provincial health education officer. A steering committee was to be formed with representatives of the Department of Community Development and any other government offices that were able to give support to the project's objectives.

The district council works departments of Luangwa and Lusaka Rural were to be responsible for well construction. The ward chairmen were to provide leadership in the wards, which were the focal points for all developments under Zambia's new decentralization policy of "power and responsibility to the people in rural areas". Africare was to provide financial, technical and logistic assistance.

The Ministry of Health expected that by completion of the project it would have determined how best to employ appropriate technology within its nationwide primary health care programme. The project was to be implemented by existing Zambian government departments and personnel, thus offering reasonable assurance that the knowledge and expertise developed would remain with those who had been involved.

The project area

Luangwa District and the eastern part of Lusaka Rural District extend over some 3750 km² and have about 30 000 inhabitants.

The project area was representative of the general rural health situation in Zambia. Although there were two mission hospitals and seven government health centres, fewer than a quarter of the population went to these institutions for medical care.

The different population distribution and settlement patterns in the two districts strongly influenced people's access to health care, and would certainly affect health education and the promotion of primary health care. The Soli of Lusaka Rural live in small, scattered villages, often in family groupings of three or four households. The Kunda and the Senga-Luse of Luangwa live in larger, compact communities, some with several hundred people, near the Luangwa river.

Water and food were the common denominators of the people's expressed needs. There were few functioning wells and boreholes in the area. Most people drew water from streams and rivers. The women spent a lot of time and effort fetching water from distant sources, and the people believed abdominal pains and diarrhoea were caused by dirty water.

The people of Luangwa and Lusaka Rural are subsistence farmers. Maize is the principal crop, although some sorghum and millet (mainly for brewing beer) are grown in Luangwa. There are patches of good soil but much of the area is hilly and heavily forested. Rainfall is normally adequate in Lusaka Rural but poor in the Luangwa valley.

Upper respiratory tract infection, malaria, diarrhoea, abdominal pains and general fevers made up the majority of complaints registered at the districts' medical facilities. Skin and eye infections were also serious problems, particularly in Luangwa.

Implementation

Project implementation depended on several factors:

— the need for the local community to understand the concept of primary health care and the various elements of health to be addressed;
— the need for community members to understand their role in planning, implementing and evaluating the project;
— the need for the individual communities to come up with a list of their needs and problems according to priorities;
— the need for each community to examine critically its limitations, in terms of capacity and resources, in addressing its needs and problems.

The first six months of the project concentrated on educating and motivating the community. The project staff and the Ministry of Health were totally convinced that the success of primary health care depended on effective use of the resources available in the project area, the most important resource being the population itself. The people in the project area had to become actively involved in all aspects of the day-to-day planning and management of primary health care project activities in their communities. The project coordinator had to open a dialogue with the community and government departments. Fortunately, the Ministry of Health had already involved chiefs and ward chairmen in seminars on primary health care in the project area.

During this process, a total of 59 meetings were held with village headmen, village health committee chairmen, ward chairmen, officials of wards, branches and district councils, and other government officials, including district executive secretaries and district governors. A further 195 visits were made to community projects and residences of community representatives. The health workers had to explain what primary health care is and what would be done during the implementation of primary health care programmes throughout the country and especially in the project area.

Local leaders subsequently held public meetings to identify community needs and problems. There were four main areas of concern:

- There was a lack of clean water sources. Existing sources were streams, rivers and unprotected wells but most of them dried up before the beginning of each rainy season. The wells were shallow and needed repairing.
- The health facilities were inaccessible to some of the communities.
- Most pregnant women avoided going to male medical staff for delivery.
- The people associated diarrhoea with poor drinking-water and lack of latrines.

Many communities resolved to construct new wells and repair or deepen old ones. Community health workers had to be selected and trained in areas that were far from existing health facilities. New rural health centre staff houses had to be built to accommodate trained health assistants and nurse-midwives, and latrines had to be built for village households.

The needs of the community, especially for construction and repair of wells, were communicated to the district councils of Luangwa and Lusaka Rural by ward chairmen. Each district council in turn submitted a list of well sites to the project coordinator.

Some 24 village health committees and six rural health centre committees were formed. Some of the village health committees were based on the political party's section committees, some were subsidiaries of village productivity committees and some were entirely new committees.

Intersectoral cooperation was fostered in both districts. The Departments of Water Affairs, Agriculture, Public Works and Education, the district councils and the Zambia National Service (for secondary school leavers) played major roles in carrying out the project.

Accomplishments

During the project's early years, the following activities were carried out:

- Seventeen community health workers successfully completed a six-week training course that included basic knowledge of agriculture and nutrition, maintenance of wells, identification of malnourished children, promotion of environmental health, diagnosis and treatment of minor ailments and community organization.
- Thirteen wells were built and two were restored. Nine wells were dug but not protected and 10 were left uncompleted.
- Six health committees were formed and three former health committees were revived. Following the formation of the health committees, 133 latrines were built and put to use by individual households. The idea of ventilated improved pit (VIP) latrines was introduced in villages, schools and rural health centres. The Social Secretary for Luangwa District wrote to all primary school head teachers urging them to adopt the VIP technology which eliminates odour and traps disease-bearing flies. The initial response was not encouraging but, as public education continued, more progress was made in schools than at the rural health centres. The schools were able to mobilize schoolchildren to make bricks, which was not the case at health centres.
- Six rural health centre staff houses were to be constructed and by the end of the first year 47 000 bricks had been either donated or moulded in self-help schemes by the communities of Rufunsa, Kasinsa and Mwantigora. At Lukwipa, the rural health centre was built as far as wall-plate level during the first year. The local response to these self-help activities varied considerably. The people in the Mwantigora rural health centre catchment area worked diligently with officers from government departments. The local community provided bricklayers and general workers at very low salaries. The women collected water and provided food while the men provided sand and gravel. The staff house was completed in late 1984. At Kasinsa, however, the people at first did not want to construct the house on a self-help basis. They agreed only after community leaders intervened, but progress proved to be very slow. Work at other sites also proceeded by fits and starts.

Evaluation

In February 1985, Africare and the Ministry of Health jointly evaluated progress over the first two and a half years. The report was critical of all parties concerned but expressed confidence that the original objectives could nevertheless be achieved. The evaluation team recommended that:

- — the project should be extended for two years;
- — responsibility for the project should be transferred from the Ministry

of Health's Primary Health Care Secretariat to the district councils, in conformity with the government's policy of decentralization;
— the project's philosophy and goals should be discussed and clarified with the district councils which should integrate the project into their district development and work plans;
— the Provincial Medical Officer's building team should help to construct the rural health centre staff houses.

Implementation, 1985–1990

As soon as both district councils had accepted basic responsibility for planning and implementing the project, the Provincial Medical Officer, in consultation with Africare, decided to reduce the area to be covered by a newly assigned project coordinator. While the latter continued to focus on Luangwa District and the water component for Lusaka Rural, another Ministry officer was appointed to handle activities of the project in Lusaka Rural District. It was hoped this would aid the project coordinator by allowing him to concentrate on a more compact area.

The project coordinator and the Provincial Medical Officer met with the key district council officials, chiefs, ward chairmen and communities. The meetings were aimed at motivating the communities and updating the list of wells to be constructed and repaired. During the meetings the district councils committed themselves to transport building materials to the project sites.

In spite of organizational changes, the project continued to experience chronic delays in achieving its objectives over the next few years. The following section summarizes accomplishments as of mid-1990 when Africare and the Ministry prepared formally to end the project.

Training of community health workers

Fifteen community health workers were trained in Luangwa District and two refresher courses were conducted for them. Lusaka Rural District trained a second set of 10 community health workers and five traditional birth attendants.

The community health workers' activities were weakened because the communities were unable to support them. Most people—especially in Luangwa—suffered persistent hunger. The community health workers in Luangwa District were constantly on the move in search of food for their families and the Christian Children's Fund, an American NGO, agreed to support them financially. In Lusaka Rural hunger was not such a serious problem but community health workers there received no support from the community or from other sources. The community health workers in both districts tended to emphasize the dispensing of drugs rather than the promotion of environmental health.

Construction and rehabilitation of wells

Because of the councils' continued failure to construct and repair wells, Africare decided to test a manually operated drilling rig which local communities could use to drill their own wells. People were eager to use the equipment but rock and other impenetrable strata limited its usefulness. Only eight wells were drilled and equipped with hand pumps before the drilling rig had to be withdrawn.

Ventilated improved pit latrines

Promotion of the ventilated improved pit latrines continued. However, villagers were reluctant to have them because of the expenses involved for cement and wire mesh for fly screens.

Construction of staff houses

With the exception of Lukwipa and Mwantigora, communities throughout the project area failed to support the building of staff housing for rural health centres. Work stretched over several years, little self-help labour was forthcoming, promised bricks were not delivered and building supplies were stranded in Lusaka for lack of transport.

Analysis of constraints

Five important assumptions made during the project design proved to be unfounded. These were:

— that the people would render their skills and labour on a self-help basis;
— that government departments operating in the project area would provide the required technical support;
— that Luangwa and Lusaka Rural district councils would transport building materials from Lusaka to the project sites;
— that, with Africare providing well moulds and cement, the Luangwa and Lusaka Rural district councils would be able to install wells with reasonable efficiency;
— that the rural health centre houses (six units in all) would be completed within the first year, thus allowing full staffing in the project area.

It was also believed that a Primary Health Care Secretariat within the Ministry of Health headquarters and the Primary Health Care Inter-sectoral Cooperation Committees which had been formed at national, provincial and district levels would aid project implementation. The secretariat and the intersectoral committees were mandated to supervise and monitor primary health care activities in the country.

Initially the spirit among health officials involved in this project was high. Primary health care meetings and workshops were held at all levels. At the start of the project, workshops were conducted for chiefs, ward chairmen and other influential community leaders.

The project coordinator was expected to reinforce the Ministry of Health's interaction with the community at district and village levels. The project coordinator's tasks were to visit community health workers and acquaint them with the programme and to meet key officials and community leaders. The coordinator was also to transport building materials from Lusaka and within the project area but the carrying capacity of the project's sole vehicle was limited.

It is worth examining each of the key assumptions in detail to learn precisely what went wrong.

Community ability to provide self-help labour

Mwantigora was the only community to finish a rural health centre staff house within two years. Although the partially completed Kasinsa rural health centre staff house was occupied by a health assistant by 1988, it had taken six years to reach that stage. The efforts of the skilled workers were not coordinated and, like the general workers, they demanded payment. As the area's economy declined, however, a number of skilled workers abandoned the work. The only bricklayer, who had kept the work going, eventually left the area in search of a more rewarding job in town.

In general, local leaders failed to mobilize the people to provide self-help labour. The extreme poverty of the area and other factors such as the lack of transport for supplies increased people's reluctance to get involved in projects about which they had not been directly consulted during planning.

Technical assistance by government departments

There was limited intersectoral cooperation among government departments. Most regarded the project as Africare's. A few departments offered some technical or material assistance but, on the whole, they were either unable or unwilling to provide necessary support. Coordination at district level was poor. Effective district and provincial leadership might have mitigated these problems, but such leadership was lacking throughout the life of the project.

Materials

Both district councils agreed to provide transport for building materials from Lusaka and within the project area but in practice this almost never happened. District council lorries were often "off the road". When they were operating, it seemed difficult for those responsible to arrange collection of building materials in Lusaka.

District councils and well construction

At the beginning of the project in September 1982, both district councils were requested to submit lists of sites at which the communities were ready to construct wells on a self-help basis. The lists were updated annually. More often than not, the district councils failed to submit the required information.

Some of the well sites recommended by the district councils were in villages where communities had expressed no need of them. Some communities went ahead digging wells without having been registered on the councils' lists. The lack of adherence to work schedules and lists of wells came about largely because of poor communication between ward chairmen and the development secretaries of the district councils. Each council was able to construct or repair only two or three wells during each dry season. The rest of the hand-dug wells collapsed during the next rainy season.

Construction of staff houses

When the project began, rural health centres in Luangwa and Lusaka Rural were inadequately staffed. There were only three health assistants to help the project coordinator in community organization and motivation. Four rural health centres had no health assistants or nurses. The planned six housing units were to enable the Ministry of Health to alleviate the staff shortage in the first year of the project. Of six houses, only one was completed within the first two years and a second house, although not completely finished, was occupied towards the end of 1987. Throughout the project, therefore, lack of adequate staffing greatly hindered the project coordinator and seriously reduced the project's level of success.

Analysis of original project design

The project was clearly too ambitious and seriously overestimated the willingness and capacity of the district councils to collaborate. Although the design team went to some length to consult with the people and community leaders, they failed to involve the Provincial Medical Officer in Lusaka. They also failed to involve the district councils and their departmental staff sufficiently in the planning process. The project that emerged was widely perceived as Africare's or the Ministry's. It was certainly not seen as a project of the people or the district councils.

A pilot project should be given a decent opportunity to demonstrate what can be achieved in an area that is more or less typical of areas where the project might be replicated. Luangwa District is perhaps one of the least typical districts in Zambia, with its large villages, poor soil, and erratic and low rainfall. Its people also showed little enthusiasm for the latrines that were to be the project's principal means to improve environmental health.

The sparsely populated eastern section of Lusaka Rural presented logistic and administrative problems. Visiting widely scattered family homesteads (unlike Luangwa's populous and compact villages) was extremely time-consuming for the project coordinator. The district council staff, who operated from two towns on opposite sides of the capital city, also found it difficult to serve this sector.

The project would probably have done better to concentrate on just one of the two districts. It would have benefited even more if it had been implemented in a district where the demographic characteristics, village structures and receptivity to new ideas were more representative of the Zambian countryside.

Even if the project had been perfectly designed for the perfect pilot area, it was burdened from the start by unclear lines of command. Normally, the Provincial Medical Officer for Lusaka Province should have participated fully in planning the project and should have taken responsibility for implementing it. In this case, the Primary Health Care Secretariat took all initiatives, under the direction of the Assistant Director of Medical Services (Planning). The Provincial Medical Officer played no part in the planning and, not surprisingly, failed to take any interest in the project's implementation. This became critical when the secretariat lost its expatriate head (who had conceived the project) and its senior Zambian officer who had served on the design team. The situation was aggravated by the departure from Zambia of Africare's resident representative, who had participated in the design of the project, one year after implementation began.

The administrative muddle was never truly resolved. In theory the Ministry should have been fully responsible for implementation, with the district councils playing an important but subordinate role. Africare's role should have been limited to monitoring, evaluation and disbursement of funds, as needed. Instead the NGO was drawn constantly, and reluctantly, into an implementing role.

The picture was further complicated by the arrival in Luangwa District, soon after the project was initiated, of another foreign NGO. The newcomer was eager to channel funds directly to villages to support development activities. It set up committees in several villages and invited them to identify needs which could be addressed with periodic infusions of cash. With access to seemingly unlimited funds, the committees chose to pay people to work on various development projects. This naturally undermined their interest in working on self-help components of the project that Africare was supporting, notably the construction of housing for clinic staff.

It can be argued that the project achieved some of its goals and that, regardless of the extended time required, it has improved the health standards in much of the target area. Unfortunately, no reliable baseline data were developed during the early years of the project. It must be taken on faith that the 32 community health workers trained, the 25 wells dug or repaired, and the introduction of latrines have had at least a modest impact. How much, we shall never know. What we can conclude, however, is that the resources devoted to the project would almost certainly have been better spent elsewhere in Zambia, under less adverse circumstances.

CHAPTER 4

Oxfam's experience of working in primary health care in the Eastern Province of Zambia

I. Birch

Background to the primary health care programme

Support for health care has always been an important part of Oxfam's work in Zambia, as elsewhere, but it has become a greater priority in recent years. Rapid and severe contraction of the Zambian economy has caused a rise in the price of essential commodities and a decline in the provision of basic services. An effective primary health care system could have a vital role in identifying those people most vulnerable to these changes.

The Zambian Ministry of Health asked Oxfam in 1985 to consider supporting its primary health care programme. Oxfam had previously worked mainly through local NGOs and community groups, and a direct working relationship with government on this scale was a new departure.

From the outset, however, the aim was neither to replace government funding nor to duplicate the activities of the major multilateral and bilateral donors. Instead, Oxfam offered an approach to primary health care shaped by the organization's philosophy and experience. The 1985–86 annual report of Oxfam's Lusaka office asked about primary health care: "Does it mean healthier people, or rather people taking more control over their own health in its widest sense? The two imply very different things, and we come down very strongly on the side of this second interpretation."

That report listed four key components felt to be vital to the success of primary health care: full involvement of the community, strong inter-sectoral links, efficient monitoring and evaluation, and adequate material support. These conclusions were drawn from Oxfam's experience of similar work in the region (for example, in the United Republic of Tanzania) and in particular from the work of the Private Hospitals Association of Malawi (PHAM), with which Oxfam has been associated since 1981. The interpretation of primary health care used in the Zambian programme is one developed by PHAM and described as "a comprehensive system of care immediately surrounding individuals where they live. This system of care is administered by the individuals themselves, by the family, by the society around them, and by others. Everyone is involved in it."

PHAM emphasized the need to train field workers from every sector, not just health, to adopt a problem-solving and open attitude. A paper prepared by PHAM in 1986 noted that "most training up to the present time has concentrated on making sure that service personnel have all the answers to the problems in a community, and therefore any failures are the failure of people in following the advice given."

The PHAM aim was to reverse this relationship between experts and the community. It is necessary to ask if everyone has equal access to a comprehensive system of health care as described above. If not, why not? And are existing structures and services relevant to people's needs, especially those families most at risk? The emphasis is on getting the approach right first and letting specific activities such as growth monitoring, immunization or water provision follow from that.

In early discussions with the Ministry of Health of Zambia it was felt that the pilot programme should be limited to Katete, Lundazi and Chipata where Oxfam had been funding nutrition and agricultural groups for several years. Oxfam's previous grassroots experience and connections in the Eastern Province strengthened its ability to make the cross-sectoral links that are an essential factor in primary health care.

Oxfam staff visited all three districts in September and December 1985 to learn about the kinds of primary health care activities already taking place and to discuss what the most appropriate form of assistance might be. The concerns expressed by each district corresponded fairly closely: lack of resources such as adequate transport and funds, lack of motivation, poor supervision, poor relationships between community health workers and their communities, and weak intersectoral cooperation. In June 1986, after reaching mutual agreement with each of the districts on the practical details of their plans, Oxfam approved a series of three-year grants.

Funds were allocated to strengthen human skills and resources through a variety of training sessions, workshops and seminars, and to meet practical programme running costs such as those for vehicles, bicycles, spare parts and fuel. In addition, grants were made for annual evaluation workshops that would measure progress in terms of mutually determined goals.

In summary, the key objectives of the Eastern Province primary health care programme were as follows:

— to improve the relationship between the primary health care system and the community, through training for primary health care workers and by increasing the involvement of the community in evaluating and planning primary health care;
— to improve intersectoral cooperation, especially at local level;
— to improve data collection, analysis and use;
— to improve logistic support, especially transport, for primary health care.

resources have all weakened that link. Poor understanding of the purpose and role of community health workers is hardly surprising since communities were not directly involved in the planning and implementation of the programme.

The limited support for community health workers (and to a lesser extent for TBAs) at village level stems from several factors. Firstly, the assumption that community health workers would be given some form of material support by their communities has proved to be false — and is now even less likely in view of the reduction in people's capacity to make voluntary donations of any kind.

Secondly, community health workers are seen by many villagers as government employees — understandably, since the government trains them and supplies them with bicycles and drugs — who should therefore be remunerated by government. This is not the role the community health workers were intended to play, nor is it their own perception of their role. But for as long as community health workers are seen as accountable to the Ministry of Health, they will not succeed in being truly accountable to their communities. Sadly, the same is happening with TBAs, whose traditional significance within the community is being eroded. In February 1987 Oxfam reported the "bizarre situation" of traditional support and reward mechanisms disappearing as a result of government intervention. "Once trained, the TBAs are regarded as 'different'," Oxfam said, adding that in many people's eyes support of trained TBAs "is no longer the function of the community but that of the government".

Thirdly, most community health workers are men. In theory they are selected by the community but in practice they are often chosen by a select group of village leaders. Since a major part of the work concerns mother and child health, this adds to their alienation.

Fourthly, the area which some community health workers have to cover is too large. Consequently many of them are working too many hours each week, to the detriment of their income and family support. In February 1987 there were 58 community health workers in Lundazi District, each covering between 5 and 10 villages and each working about 40 hours a week with little financial or other support. The average catchment population for community health workers in Chipata District for the same period was between 1500 and 2000 people.

Lastly, the status of community health workers is further eroded if their supply of drugs runs out. Villagers lose confidence in them and may bypass them completely. Katete's report for the year ending June 1990 noted that, although the supply of drugs to rural health centres was good, there were no extra stocks with which to equip community health workers. "A simple curative stock would greatly assist the promotion of health issues by these workers," the report said.

The district teams in Lundazi and Chipata have even discussed removing the curative role of the community health workers. This has had to be balanced, however, against the danger of damaging community support still further and adding to confusion about the role of the community health workers.

These problems are common to all three districts and have been addressed in different ways. Katete has done two things. Firstly, the district has minimized the level of formal training given to TBAs. Instead of formal government-run courses, each TBA is visited at home by family health nurses. This has helped to support the perception of the TBA as part of the existing village tradition and it has encouraged people to continue making use of TBA skills.

The role of TBAs is increasingly significant. Five years ago the surveys undertaken by the Lundazi nutrition group revealed that 83.8% of women were giving birth at home. Now though, with the advent of hospital charges and higher costs for transport, the proportion of women giving birth in the village, including those giving birth for the first time and those most at risk, is increasing even further. Katete has proposed greater attention to TBA training since delivery rates in rural health centres and hospitals went down substantially after fees were introduced. The consequent effect on the workload and psychological stress of TBAs can be considerable. One was quoted as saying of women in labour, "I have no choice. When they are in an advanced stage, I have to deliver them here and bear the consequences."

Katete has also begun to experiment with a new kind of community-level health worker — the village health volunteer. The first group of 16 village health volunteers began their training in the Vulamokoko area in August 1987. By early 1989 there were 22 in action in the district, about half of them women. Village health volunteers are trained in a small number of skills such as growth monitoring of children under five and the recognition of common diseases. The volunteers are given a weighing scale but no drugs or bicycle since their catchment area is their own village. In theory, therefore, the system of village health volunteers removes some of the problems of the community health worker structure. The village volunteers have smaller areas and populations to cover, no transport problems, closer acquaintance with communities and more clearly defined roles.

Another benefit of this scheme has become apparent. Several parts of Katete were seriously affected by the war in Mozambique which periodically spilled across the border. Health centres were a particular target. The centre at Kafumbwe was attacked three times and closed for one and a half years. Some community health workers stopped travelling to war-affected areas but the local village health volunteers were able to reduce the damage caused by their absence.

Moving responsibility for an activity such as growth monitoring to village level has the potential to raise the community's sense of "ownership" of that activity. While the weighing of children under five years of age was formerly the responsibility of the rural health centre, with the results centralized there or at district level, under the new village health volunteer scheme the responsibility for gathering information is clearly within the village itself. The nutrition surveys carried out in Katete from 1986 to 1988 noted that "growth monitoring is vital in the development of primary health care, because it promotes the quest for knowledge and empowers communities to protect their own health".

It is perhaps too soon to tell whether or not such empowerment is really taking place, although there is some evidence that the coverage of children under five years of age is increasing. The numbers attending monthly monitoring in the Vulamokoko area between January and December 1988 ranged from 1700 to 2800—an average of 56% of a target population of 4000. Corresponding figures for 1987 in the same area averaged 25%.

Nevertheless, there are problems with the village health volunteer scheme. People still expect the volunteers to give out drugs, and there is some disappointment when they don't. There are obvious difficulties caused by the addition of another tier of community worker. Confusion arises between the roles of community health workers and village health volunteers and because of overlap with the child monitoring being carried out by the immunization outreach team from St Francis Hospital. There has also been a failure to involve the most vulnerable families in the design and implementation of the project, despite discussions with villagers. The Katete team has acknowledged the difficulty of measuring the effectiveness of village discussions and is now considering using household surveys to assess progress.

Another way the team is attempting to bridge the gap with the community is by carrying out a health survey in 24 villages. The aim is "to establish basic health data for rural communities over a three-year period so that future health planning can be evolved to respond to village needs." The surveys will be carried out monthly by a community health worker or a village health volunteer with regular supervisory visits by the Primary Health Care Coordinator. Each year there will be an evaluation seminar for feedback and future planning. The effectiveness of such a programme remains to be seen but it demonstrates a welcome commitment to start the planning of district programmes from village-based needs upwards. The team in Lundazi chose a different response to the same problem of poor community participation. The team began a series of motivation seminars aimed at bringing community members together to discuss issues related to primary health care and to work out possible solutions to problems faced by the programme. Twenty-four seminars had been held by the end of 1989. Many of the seminars were followed up in succeeding months by visits from the primary health care team so that the effect of these meetings on problems such as support for community health workers might be monitored.

Despite this initiative, the Lundazi team still faced the problem of how to involve a true cross-section of the community—not just the (mostly male) village leaders, but those whom the leaders were supposed to represent. It seems that none of the district teams have found an effective way around this problem, although many of their ideas (such as devolving growth monitoring to village level) are steps in the right direction.

Intersectoral cooperation

During a development workshop in Zambia's Eastern Province in May 1990, participants used role-play to demonstrate the confusion that can occur when development projects are not coordinated. An account of the role-play read as follows:

> The agricultural officer visits the women's club to ask them to go for a field day at one of the fields in the villages. As the women prepare to leave, the social development assistant also appears and requests the same club members to start their functional literacy lessons. All of a sudden the health assistant also appears requesting the same women to bring all under-five children to the clinic. The nutrition demonstrator arrives shortly to carry out a cooking demonstration lesson. Finally the party ward chairman comes to inform the women that they were requested to prepare for the ward council, and disperses the women since time had run out.

The role-play was of course hypothetical but it nicely demonstrates the problems that can arise when there is a lack of cooperation and coordination between community and extension workers in the same area. The workshop report demonstrated clearly the ways that different sectors overlap. The Eastern Province primary health care programme was built on the premise that primary health care is not solely a health issue but also requires active cooperation of other departments whose work has a direct or indirect impact on the health status of the population.

Current government structures impede effective intersectoral activity. Education, health and social development are the responsibility of the Social Secretary, while the Department of Works and the Department of Agriculture remain the responsibility of the Development Secretary. The inflexibility of a formal bureaucratic structure means that departments tend to run programmes in isolation. All three districts identified at an early stage that the lack of coordination was a major weakness of primary health care in the province. They have tried to address this problem in several ways.

In Chipata, an intersectoral primary health care committee was organized. It was the second of its kind in Zambia and described its purpose as "to coordinate the activities of other departments so as to attain a unified or uniform community approach". At its meeting of 5 November 1987, the Chipata intersectoral committee "strongly deplored the individualistic stands that government departments have been using in approaching the rural communities. Such individualistic stands have not been of benefit to the community."

The first objective of the Chipata committee was to strengthen interdisciplinary cooperation in two pilot areas, Mpomwa and Chanje. The district team and local extension workers visited Mpomwa and Chanje every two weeks. Their aim, according to the District Social Development Officer, was "to find out from people what their problems are, since we can't identify problems for them".

The eventual aim was to have multisectoral teams at village/area level, and by June 1988 there were five. These were visited each month by representatives of the district primary health care team who also followed up specific requests. For example, three areas requested help with water supply. The district team discussed this with the relevant authorities in Chipata and then obtained agreement to help with shallow wells. Nevertheless, the intersectoral committee noticed that some departments were reluctant to support these pilot initiatives fully. The committee therefore began a series of workshops so the problem could be discussed both at district level and in the pilot areas.

The district team certainly tried to find ways around problems. However, clear evidence of the practical impact of these initiatives is lacking. Reports contain comments such as "coverage increased" or "support improved", but there is no statistical information to substantiate this. Chipata is not alone in this respect.

Lundazi already enjoyed excellent cooperation between sectors through the work of the nutrition group. The regular field days in Lundazi involved health, nutrition and agriculture personnel in a varied programme of discussions, demonstrations and drama. Building on the work of the nutrition group, the Lundazi primary health care team ran a series of intersectoral seminars across the district. These had several purposes, one of the key ones being to facilitate discussions between participants and resource personnel in order to get a picture of real needs.

The seminars were attended by community leaders, traditional chiefs, head teachers, agricultural assistants and district health personnel. By December 1989, 15 had been held in various locations. The Lundazi report for the year ending 1989 commented that one aim behind the seminars was "to minimise interdepartmental conflicts by creating friendship and the desire to work together". This is a positive idea but again there is little of substance to show how far it has been achieved or what impact it has had on work at local level.

The work of the nutrition group and the introduction of intersectoral seminars were informal ways of encouraging cooperation. However, a formal structure to promote intersectoral cooperation at district level was the District Primary Health Care Committee, which held its first meeting in its newly resurrected state in January 1988. The meeting was attended by staff from various departments and was chaired by the

District Governor. This was crucial, since lack of support from senior government personnel had been identified as the main reason why such groups had failed in the past.

The minutes of that meeting showed that the committee was promising changes in the right directions. However, the committee did not meet at all during 1989. Without effective support at senior levels, efforts such as those in Chipata and Lundazi to encourage integration across sectors will remain isolated ones.

The examples from the two districts illustrate the changing relationship between the district team and the community, with a welcome shift of emphasis and attitude from that of teacher to that of learner. The change of approach is being wrought against the pressures bequeathed by generations of top–down tuition.

All these initiatives — village health volunteers, intersectoral teams, motivation seminars — may or may not have strengthened primary health care in the province. A detailed assessment of their impact has yet to be carried out. But the fact that district staff have identified problems in their work and have thought through some possible solutions is a significant development. Readiness to learn from experience, to experiment with new ideas and to step outside customary limits is an illustration of precisely the kind of personal development that the primary health care programme aimed to encourage.

The Primary Health Care Coordinating Committee

As the three-year pilot programme progressed, district staff played a more active role in discussions with Oxfam and with government. An example of their growing self-awareness was the creation of the Primary Health Care Coordinating Committee which developed from the annual evaluation workshop in Chipata in March 1990, and which has provided a forum for discussion of a range of issues, including future support.

The purpose of this committee is to coordinate primary health care programmes in the member districts and facilitate exchange among them (for example, through the circulation of reports and newsletters, or through interdistrict visits). The second meeting of the Primary Health Care Coordinating Committee proposed that Petauke District also be represented. Petauke was the only district in the province not already a member since Chama and Chadiza districts, although receiving no direct funding from Oxfam, had been associated with the programme for several years through attendance at workshops and visits from programme staff.

One of the motivating factors behind the creation of the coordinating committee was the recognition by delegates that primary health care structures dominated by one sector (health) were limiting the scope and delivery of services. There were signs that other departments (education, agriculture and so on) were feeling left out, and Oxfam was seen as being managed by health service employees. Twelve members were elected to the first Primary Health Care Coordinating Committee, with representatives from the health sector still outnumbering others three to one. Despite the continued imbalance, recognition of the problem is itself an important development.

Another impetus behind the creation of the Primary Health Care Coordinating Committee was the districts' frustration at the slow-moving bureaucracy of a centralized Ministry. Delays in the receipt of funds, routed via the Primary Health Care Secretariat in Lusaka to the districts, have been a problem since the programme began. The Primary Health Care Coordinating Committee will have its own bank account to which the Ministry has agreed that funds may be transferred directly by donors.

The creation of the coordinating committee also demonstrates a growing willingness on the part of the district teams to work together, a greater awareness of the need for mutual accountability, and a readiness to learn from and monitor each other's programmes. At the 1990 evaluation workshop each district plan was presented to the participants, who recorded their dissatisfaction with one of them and asked that it be presented again the next day. The workshop report records that "no mention was made of the constraints which might have been encountered by the primary health care team. The house wondered if this was because there were no constraints at all or if this was just an omission."

Another district was asked why it had decided to expand a pilot project before problems that had arisen in its initial stages had been addressed. The meeting also felt that none of the district reports were acceptable as evaluation reports, and asked a small group to meet with the Provincial Medical Officer to work out some guidelines and a format which the districts could then use to rewrite their reports.

There is also evidence of a readiness to challenge directives which members feel are inappropriate to their work. An instruction from the Provincial Medical Officer to form another coordinating committee for the Universal Child Immunization programme "was felt to be unfair ... when after all the UCI was a component to primary health care".

The Primary Health Care Coordinating Committee is a new development which may also bring problems of its own. The former approach was to operate inside existing ministerial structures, attempting to influence from within. The creation of a committee outside those structures may lead to its work being marginalized. Nevertheless, the innovation is welcome and Oxfam will watch its development with interest.

Conclusion

At the end of this first period of support the three districts are, together with Oxfam, trying to review progress and identify areas that need more discussion and attention. Some conclusions can be drawn from this experience which are of particular concern to an NGO such as Oxfam.

Firstly, the programme's emphasis on training and on the development of new approaches and skills is a logical one, but there is an obvious danger of concentrating attention too narrowly and of failing to ensure that such skills are spread widely enough. One could argue that new ideas and experience will gradually permeate the system, passing from one individual and team to another. In view of the high turnover rates within districts, however, the continuity needed for this to happen cannot be guaranteed.

Secondly, it is still not clear whether reorienting the approach of one part of a much larger bureaucratic network is a realistic aim for an NGO with relatively little muscle to flex (even if muscle-flexing by NGOs were desirable). Changes have certainly been seen in the district teams in the programme but how far these changes might be replicated elsewhere is unknown. The Primary Health Care Secretariat in Lusaka has in the past welcomed the Oxfam-funded programme as a vehicle for trying out new ideas, but the logical extension of those ideas challenges the system to work in radically different ways.

This in turn raises the issue of sustainability and the question of how far large-scale reliance on external support is a realistic option for the health sector. Perhaps the kind of approach advocated in this programme — one which concentrates on strengthening resources that are already available — will prove in the long term to be the most viable. Even so, Oxfam found itself being slowly sucked into the apparently bottomless pit of health-sector funding. The demand for more is always there, and with it the danger that Oxfam's ability to maintain its own priorities and parameters could gradually be eroded as needs increase.

The primary health care programme has placed great demands not only on Oxfam's financial resources but also on the capacity of the organization's staff in Zambia to service the programme. Oxfam's links with partner agencies are enriching but time-consuming. The primary health care work in the Eastern Province is but one part of a much wider network of Oxfam support throughout the country, and it has to compete with equally pressing demands on the time and resources of the organization's staff.

In Zambia's current economic environment this work requires much more analytical and qualitative data and more accurate targeting of risk groups. In a situation of growing needs and diminishing capacity to meet them, it is essential that remaining resources are put to the best possible use. Despite the progress made, the ability to gather and use information to the best advantage has consistently eluded the Eastern Province primary health care teams. Lack of qualitative analysis makes it difficult to evaluate the strengths and weaknesses of the programme. This must therefore be a major objective of any future proposals.

Despite the fact that the work has been carried out in conjunction with the Ministry of Health, it has never been treated as specifically a "health" programme. This is not simply because primary health care is more than just a health issue. It is also because the principles that underly the programme and the approach adopted throughout are exactly the same as those used by Oxfam elsewhere in Zambia. The ultimate aim has been one of empowerment and a reversal of existing roles and responsibilities. Such an approach takes time and can be flawed. Ultimately, however, it throws down a challenge to those with power — whether it is the power of information, or of skills, or of policy-making, or of funding. The challenge is to allow others to share in that power and benefit from it.

CHAPTER 5

The Kaputa experience: antecedents of primary health care

J. Macdonald

Joint approaches

Like many countries in Africa, Zambia has adopted the principles of primary health care as the most rational strategy for tackling the urgent health problems of its population. Also, as in all countries of the world, it took some time in Zambia before primary health care was taken seriously as an alternative approach to the provision of health care. The success of the approach will be a more effective health care system but if this is to come about we have to learn from past achievements and failures. The experience in Kaputa in the 1970s reflects some of the difficulties inherent in the primary health care approach as well as its potential for promoting the well-being of the population. The Kaputa experience was certainly not the only antecedent of the primary health care approach in Zambia but it was an effort to move towards a primary health care approach even before the formulations of the International Conference on Primary Health Care in Alma-Ata in 1978.

Primary health care tackles the most common diseases of a country, provides a system of referral for serious cases, and promotes health and prevents disease where possible. The Alma-Ata conference was clear about these aims, as is the Government of Zambia. According to the Declaration of Alma-Ata, referred to in the Preface, primary health care "addresses the main health problems in the community, providing promotive, preventive, curative and rehabilitative services accordingly".

The Government of Zambia echoed this in its 1980 final document on primary health care which is referred to by Kasonde & Martin in Chapter 2. That document called primary health care "a practical approach to making essential health care universally accessible to individuals and families in the community in an acceptable and affordable way and with their full participation".

In order to meet these aims, primary health care has several targets. These are often called the "elements" of primary health care. These targets include improving the nutritional status of the population, especially children under five years of age, training and deploying appropriate levels of care providers such as community health workers, educating people about preventable diseases, and providing a safe and adequate water supply. These are important aims but more important perhaps in terms of the challenge to the health services are the strategies for meeting these aims. Strategies basic to primary health care are a multisectoral approach and involvement by the community. These two strategies, though easy to understand in themselves, are not so easy to put into practice. The different sectors are not used to working together in a coordinated manner, the health sector is not equipped to lead in this direction and its efforts to provide leadership are in any case not always appreciated by the other sectors. Communities, on the other hand, are rarely used to being significantly involved in decision-making, yet research—and indeed common sense—shows this to be the most important part of participation. Participation in carrying bricks or water to execute projects other people have decided are for their benefit is a form of involvement the poor have known for a long time but is not the significant form of people's participation called for by the principles of primary health care. Most health services in developing countries are already overstretched and underfunded. Asking these services to find additional initiative, skills and energy for multisectoral collaboration and the promotion of people's participation is sometimes asking almost more than they can manage. Many of these challenges were faced, with various degrees of success, by the experiment in Kaputa.

The area now known as the Kaputa District of Zambia was, until the 1960s, remote and sparsely populated. Kaputa is in the far north of the country, bordering Zaire and Lake Tanganyika. Several seasons of heavy flooding in Kaputa brought about the creation of Lake Mweru Wantipa which proved to be extremely fertile in fish. The other lakes in Zambia, such as Bangweolu and Mweru, as well as lakes in neighbouring countries, were largely depleted through overfishing so Kaputa saw a sudden influx of people intent on making a living from the fish trade. Though no exact figures are available and fishing populations are notorious for fluctuation, the population jumped from a few thousand to perhaps 35 000. Lake Mweru Wantipa became Zambia's single largest source of protein.

The population of Kaputa was far from homogeneous, family life was often disrupted and there was no traditional sense of pride in belonging to an area. The health problems were numerous. Cholera was suspected in at least one of the fishing camps in the early 1970s. Living conditions were poor.

Kaputa was ripe for primary health care. The administrative district had recently been formed, with most of the government sectors starting work in the area around the lake which was the heart of the district. There were three government health centres but no district hospital. Historically the churches had played a role in the provision of health care in rural Zambia but this was not the case in Kaputa since church structures were only just beginning to take shape there. The relevance of this will become immediately obvious, since one aspect of the Kaputa project was to challenge all potential providers of health care—and indeed development—whether governmental, nongovernmental or church, to work together in an integrated way (hence the name Kaputa Joint Development Project). The project aimed to meet the basic health needs of the community by making best use of the available resources of the district. The assumption was that every district already has the basic resources, whether governmental or nongovernmental, to improve the quality of life in the area. The task is often to link needs, know-how and resources. By trying to implement the principles of primary health care—a multisectoral approach and the participation of the community—the Kaputa project was an effort to meet health needs by using the available professional and community-based resources. The project's statement of purpose described the project as "an integrated development project, drawing on Government, Party and Church resources to animate the self-development of people living in villages and fishing camps of the Kaputa District".

Integration was an important element of the Kaputa project. It was a serious attempt to implement the principle of multisectoral collaboration. All agencies, government or other, with a professed concern for the development and well-being of the inhabitants of the district were invited to work, not parallel to one another or indeed in rivalry, but as a team. Community participation was also encouraged. In the villages there already existed "village development committees" that had been set up by the government for the express purpose of two-way communication between government structures and the rural communities. These committees were chosen to be the usual community link in the Kaputa project. It has to be said that these committees were largely inactive, but the project took the view that the programme could be a means of revitalizing them by giving them a clearer purpose and by offering them support. The intention was to have in Kaputa District a model of health and development which could be replicated in any district of the country (there were at that time more than 50 districts). Accordingly, the emphasis was not to be on outside intervention and help. Rather, the intention was to maximize local governmental and nongovernmental professional help, plus the resources of the community itself.

There were several months of preparation of both partners in this venture (the government and church workers on one hand and the communities of the district on the other). During the phase of pre-programme education, interested villages were each invited to choose two persons for training as community health workers. At that time (1976) the name chosen was "community welfare workers" in order to try from the outset to eliminate the notion that these persons would be health workers in the narrow sense of medical workers. They were given basic training for six weeks with promises of further sessions later to update their knowledge and skills. Prior to this an attempt was made to help district health and development professionals acquire teaching skills through sessions to train the trainers. The content of the courses was similar to most community health worker training curricula. It included simple curative care but put strong emphasis on education and prevention. The community welfare workers were to be trained and supported by the district authorities and were to be supplied with the simplest of drugs. Their remuneration, however, was to be the responsibility of the village productivity committee. Inevitably, high expectations were laid on these community welfare workers both by government services and by the communities themselves.

Evaluation

As in so many such ventures, no evaluation was built into the Kaputa programme. Nevertheless, in 1980, more than four years after the first community welfare workers started, a participatory evaluation was carried out. Its conclusions can serve as sufficient commentary on what was by any standards an interesting experience.

A group of Kaputa villages were asked to comment on the progress of the programme. Each community was asked the same set of questions at open meetings attended by the village committees and anyone else who wished. The questions were discussed at length in open sessions and each village was asked to appoint a spokesperson to summarize the community's response. In this way a collective answer was worked out and communicated to the district organizers.

"Have you achieved the things you wanted to when you started this work?" "What are the problems now facing the work?" "How can it advance in your village?" The general purpose of these and other questions was to help the communities express how much they felt they were involved in the programme and how much they felt it had achieved.

The overall tone of the responses showed that villagers felt they had worked hard to build centres and support community workers, but that they would give up if the government did not match their efforts. For example, to the question "Have you achieved the things you set out to achieve?" one village responded, "Yes, they [our aims] have been achieved and we have paid the worker. Before people said, 'They will fail', but we have achieved them." Another village replied, "Yes, they have been achieved. We have built the small house [dispensary], we pay the worker, but the cholera brought us down." As regards problems, one village was eloquent: "The problem is the money of the worker. We pay our worker little by little. We shouted in this village for months, for a year and now for another year. It's always the same; the money still comes from our pockets—there is the real problem. We thought the government has brought us a little light; in the future the government will bring us a bigger light than this one." There were problems of high expectations, of failed promises, of poverty and of sheer fatigue. On the positive side, many villages gave clear evidence of having learned to work together and expressed pride in having achieved results through their own efforts.

As regards the aims of the programme, my personal opinion is that many were met. Cholera did hit the region and arguably would have ravaged the population even more if some primary health care structures had not been in place. Perhaps for the first time, community groups were offered some genuine framework for participation, even (in a modest way) in decision-making. Health workers had their first experience of dealing with this sort of involvement by the people. There was a real opportunity for collaboration between government, district authorities and church workers with development roles. Existing structures, such as the District Development Committee, were used to try to make some modest intersectoral collaboration a reality. Both participation and intersectoral collaboration were present in Kaputa District during this time.

One of the lessons learned is that health and development workers need training to promote genuine participation or they find it threatening. When people find a voice, health workers must be ready to listen, to support them and to sustain their involvement. Training and support are also vital for intersectoral collaboration. The hope that this integration could include churches and other NGOs was perhaps too optimistic. Collaboration between churches and the government, and between the churches themselves, in the promotion of people's health in the district virtually collapsed after some years. Another lesson was that integration requires sustained support and commitment from the top. In their evaluation the villages highlighted the problem that has been addressed in many academic papers since—the remuneration of village workers will always be problematic, especially in situations of poverty. Moreover, both government and community often expect too much of such workers. Enormous support is required for village-based workers.

Certainly for the community workers and the communities involved, this early experience in Kaputa District was a learning one, with both positive and negative lessons. Perhaps the most important lesson we learned is that primary health care is possible but that it can be very difficult to achieve.

CHAPTER 6

Community involvement in AIDS care and prevention in a rural hospital

M. Malama

It was towards the end of 1986 that patients at Chikankata Hospital were first diagnosed as infected with the human immunodeficiency virus (HIV). That year, 37 patients were found to be HIV-positive. By the end of 1987, the number had risen to 183.

A funding agency offered finance to renovate old hospital buildings and convert them into a hospice for people with HIV-related illness. The hospital did not feel, however, that this was an appropriate way to handle the problem since it was forecast that the acquired immunodeficiency syndrome (AIDS) would overwhelm established medical systems. An alternative approach to the care of patients with AIDS had to be explored.

Chikankata Hospital, which is run by the Salvation Army, is situated in a rural part of Zambia's Southern Province. The government pays some of the running costs and most employees are civil servants on government salaries. However, a number of donor agencies provide support in paying some salaries and in financing some projects.

The hospital's catchment area has a population of between 80 000 and 100 000. In 1989 there were 29 867 outpatient attendances and 8147 inpatient admissions.

The preventive and promotional programmes of the hospital cover a broad spectrum of services both within the hospital and in the surrounding district. The Primary Health Care Department is reputed to be one of the best in the country. Its activities include growth monitoring, oral rehydration therapy, encouragement of breast-feeding, immunization, family planning, women's health education, and treatment and prevention of malaria.

The Primary Health Care Department has more than 20 health centres. It trains and supervises community health workers and traditional birth attendants (TBAs). By the end of 1989, 56 community health workers and seven TBAs had been trained. There is also a school health programme with a health educator responsible for education on AIDS.

During the rainy season, when malaria and malnutrition are prevalent, the hospital is often overcrowded with some patients on "floor beds".

It was agreed that the primary health care principle of decentralized care should apply in the care of patients with AIDS. However, the existing primary health care structure was already overloaded with many other activities. AIDS was urgent and deserved a separate unit to focus on it.

It was also felt that AIDS needed special skills of education and counselling about very personal aspects of people's lives. AIDS workers would constantly have to deal with grief in families and communities. The community at large seemed to be potentially at risk.

The home-based care unit

It was therefore decided to set up a home-based care unit comprising a physician, a nurse, a social worker and a driver. The unit's tasks were threefold: to assess the needs of the patient at home and provide for those needs where possible and appropriate; to assess educational impact on the patient both in the hospital and between successive visits at home; and to trace contacts.

The team was guided in its approach by four basic assumptions:

— that patients prefer to stay at home;
— that the family is a source of strength and support for both the patient and the hospital;
— that decentralization is the best way of providing the patient with support, whether medical, nursing, social, psychological or spiritual;
— that provision of care in the community facilitates education for the family and the whole community.

Zambians usually become involved in caring for family members who are ill. Patients are not abandoned when in hospital but family members are usually at their side, giving much-needed help to hospital staff. The community is familiar with sickness, disease and death.

The strategy for management of AIDS has four phases: diagnosis and counselling, planned discharge, home-based care, and hospital care for the seriously ill who will benefit from it.

Patients are tested mainly on clinical suspicion, and if the result is positive the doctor or social worker spends time breaking the news. The patient is encouraged to inform a relative. Most patients do not hesitate and the first to know is usually the person who has been caring for them.

Once the family is involved, discharge to home-based care is discussed as an option. Most patients prefer to be visited at home rather than have to pay visits to the hospital. Those who decide against home-based care are encouraged to attend the clinics that are held twice a week in the hospital's outpatient department.

To begin with, the AIDS home-based care team went out once a week and visited most of the patients each month. The number of trips has grown to three a week as the number of patients has increased.

The original home-based care unit has now become a department with units or programmes for health education, counselling, nursing management within the hospital, pastoral care, and administration and research as well as home-based care. A project manager has been employed to coordinate the different activities of the department and there is strong emphasis on an interdisciplinary approach. The departmental head is a medical officer. All but two members of the department also have responsibilities in other parts of the hospital which helps maintain a balance that relieves the stress of working full time with AIDS patients. Those who do work full time in the department have clerical tasks as part of their job to give them relief from constant patient contact.

All the field workers in the programme are Zambian nationals as it is essential that counsellors and carers have an understanding of community attitudes and practices. All have received training in counselling.

The home-based care unit is now headed by a clinical officer. The other permanent members of the team are a nurse and a school educator, plus a driver. From time to time other members of the department may accompany the unit on visits.

The health education unit, which is headed by an educator, is responsible for coordinating all aspects of the programme related to education or training. Each month the unit holds AIDS management seminars that train health workers from Zambia and from other countries in the region, such as Botswana, Kenya, Malawi, Uganda and the United Republic of Tanzania.

The health education unit teaches the theory and practice of clinical nursing care for patients at home, as well as educational principles for AIDS education, personal counselling, community counselling and pastoral care. Administrative training focuses on record-keeping, data collection, project-writing and team-building skills.

Funding has been received to cover the cost of training in-country health groups that come for the one-week training seminars. It is the task of the health educator to keep the donors informed about the courses, while financial reporting is the responsibility of the project manager.

The counselling programme is responsible not only for coordinating counselling of patients and their families but also for training counsellors at the hospital, for coordinating the community counselling programme and for training community counsellors.

A ward is currently being built for the intensive care of patients who would benefit from hospital care. The registered nurse (a former hospital matron) who will be responsible for managing the ward is currently training ward auxiliaries to help her. For the moment, they are working in the tuberculosis ward which has a number of HIV-positive patients at any one time.

A typical day for the home-based care team starts at 7:30 when they pick up their packed lunch from the hospital kitchen. This is usually bread, eggs and tea. Sometimes local farmers who are supportive of the programme have provided supplements of meat, chicken or cheese. The team then travels to the home of the first patient. The welcome that most patients accord the team members surprises many. They are offered chairs or mats to sit on as they examine the patient and provide counselling to the whole family. The clinical officer (or nurse) examines the patient physically and asks about his or her condition since the last visit. The nurse talks to the person looking after the patient (the primary care giver), asks about problems that may have arisen and tries to answer questions. If medicines are needed, the clinical officer prescribes these and the nurse measures them out, making sure the primary care giver understands instructions about dosage. The patient's understanding of AIDS is checked and reinforced, especially if the patient is newly diagnosed. Results of blood tests of the spouse or children may be given at this stage. The use of condoms to protect an uninfected marriage partner is discussed where relevant.

The team carries food supplements that have been donated for AIDS patients and distributes these where there is a clear need. A similar donation of blankets has since diminished. Other family members who may need medical advice take advantage of such visits to seek assistance. While this is going on, the school educator engages the children in discussion about AIDS. The team visits about seven or eight patients and their families each day.

The benefits of home-based care are many. It frees much-needed hospital beds so that other programmes of care can continue to develop. The nurses and doctors have more time for the patients in the hospital. Other resources such as food and bedlinen are adequate for the remaining patients.

Since its inception, the programme has shown that the family is a source of strength both for the patient and for the hospital. The families have not rejected family members with AIDS but have cared for them despite believing that this might involve great personal risk. Home-based care continues to place heavy burdens on women in Africa who already have many other burdens to bear.

Education is more than information through the written or spoken word. Unless that information is received, retained and applied, education has not taken place. The AIDS team uses counselling to help close the gap between information transmission and application. Education takes place within the context of counselling.

As the presence of AIDS became more evident in the communities where the team was operating, questions and fears began to be expressed. Could one catch AIDS by sharing eating utensils or by caring for a person with the disease? Was AIDS a real threat to everyone?

Hadn't such symptoms been around for as long as the community could remember?

Community counselling

The team's initial meetings with a few communities or with community leaders have now developed into a process called community counselling where the principles of individual counselling are applied to whole communities. The aim of community counselling is to empower communities not only to cope with caring for patients but also to fight the AIDS epidemic through prevention and control.

Community counselling promotes the idea that the community itself—rather than specific people such as health personnel—is responsible for changing the behaviour of its members. Just as in personal counselling, community counselling follows the stages of building relationships, exploring problems, understanding, making decisions and taking action.

A positive relationship must exist between the counselling team and the community. Where a relationship of trust does not exist prior to the intervention, the counselling team must work on this as the first step in the process.

During the stage of problem exploration the team uses the skills of reflective listening, paraphrasing and summarizing to bring community members to an understanding of the problem and how they perceive it. In this case the problem is HIV infection. As in any counselling situation, understanding arises out of exploring the problem. As soon as the client (or community) has a clear perspective, decisions can be made to deal with the problem at hand. The community is thus enabled to make decisions about the problem of HIV/AIDS.

Decisions about strategies to deal with the problem of AIDS in the community will characterize what action is taken. The role of the counsellor is to act as a sounding board for the community, and a resource where necessary, through skills of reflective listening. Two counsellors have regular counselling sessions with communities.

Just as an individual initially reacts to bad news with denial, so communities go through the same process. (It is well known that most, if not all, countries were eager to blame other countries for having introduced the disease.) Progress may be slow to begin with. The client will not move on to the next stage unless convinced that a problem exists.

A community is defined as an organized structure that has the characteristics of a group—including identity and shared values—and has the capacity for effective communication on subjects affecting both personal and corporate concerns in the context of acknowledged mutual responsibility.

The most common type of community is the village. However, it is felt that similarities exist within other types of communities, making them suitable for community counselling. These similarities include the presence of leadership to which members are loyal, experience in decision-making by consensus and a sense of belonging by members to the whole.

The team works with four types of community: those based on kinship (such as villages), those based on occupation (such as farming cooperatives), those based on religion (such as churches) and those based on the political party system.

Community counselling can become a viable means of preventing HIV infection where consensus decisions are made about the organization of the community. The counselling process depends, however, on there being patients in the community.

Data collected over one year of counselling with 10 communities show that each community clearly defined what it considered were risk behaviours. The most commonly identified risk behaviours were premarital sex, unfaithfulness in marriage, indiscriminate sex when drunk and ritual cleansing by sexual intercourse (during which the widow of a dead man is cleansed or set free from the spirit of the deceased by sexual intercourse).

The communities also identified behavioural goals that they would have to achieve to eliminate the risk of HIV infection. The most commonly identified behavioural goals were faithfulness in marriage, abstinence from sex until marriage and abolition of ritual cleansing by sexual means.

The communities each came up with strategies that would help them accomplish their goals. Although all communities clearly understood that AIDS is transmitted sexually and also understood that they ought to modify their behaviour, not every community was convinced it was capable of change. Strategies adopted by communities included:

— training community members as an information resource;
— abolishing ritual cleansing by sexual means;
— giving health talks at village level;
— giving health talks to children;
— establishing a church, adopting a Christian lifestyle;
— discussing the reinstatement of marriage ceremonies as they had previously existed.

Faithfulness in marriage was listed as a goal for behaviour change in one community but no actual strategy was designed to achieve it. Another community decided to re-implement premarital counselling and traditional marriage ceremonies as a strategy for achieving faithfulness in marriage. In several communities some stages of the process have required modified strategies by the AIDS team.

Counselling communities takes time. The counsellors not only have to listen to what the community is saying but also have to sense what individuals in the community are feeling. Counsellors have to avoid decisions being made by only a few people. In any group there will be traditional leaders whose authority derives from birth or position, opinion leaders whose authority may have been earned, and people who naturally have a dominant personality. These can all be very helpful if they are going in the right direction. They can slow down progress if they have their own agendas or if they have missed the point. The counsellors have a huge task.

In the AIDS-affected areas, meetings sometimes fail to take place because there are more pressing issues for the community to deal with, such as funerals. These are very important social events. Since the counselling meetings are mostly held outdoors, the rain may also prevent or interrupt them.

Counsellors found that traditional leaders were eager to work on strategies for change and that women were highly motivated to participate in a process that would preserve their communities against AIDS. They found communities enthusiastic and committed in consensus decision-making to fight AIDS.

Conclusion

Chikankata Hospital has been a pioneer in home care and community involvement—both important elements of comprehensive care for persons with HIV/AIDS and their families. Although AIDS casts a shadow over the lives of many, the families and communities in Chikankata were ready to do what they could to fight the disease. They cared for their loved ones, and they examined traditional attitudes and practices that were contributing to the spread of AIDS. They acknowledged that AIDS was more than an individual matter.

Health and health behaviour are rooted in society. Even individual behaviour is to a large extent determined by the norms of a community. For the health status of people to change, social, economic and even cultural adjustments may have to be made. The task of the medical system should be to bring the problem to the attention of communities and facilitate the process by which communities examine, diagnose and prescribe a cure that will work for them.

In Chikankata the concept of home care for AIDS patients was developed out of necessity. Primary health care activities were overburdened so home care was developed as a parallel outreach initiated by the hospital. While the number of patients visited was small, a foundation of community confidence and mutual respect was laid. This formed the basis of community involvement. Gradually a sense of community responsibility and "ownership" of the HIV/AIDS problem was created. Constant interaction between hospital staff and community leaders led to important changes in social norms regarding sexual behaviour. As a result the communities abandoned the ritual cleansing of widows by sexual means. This change is reminiscent of the village awareness-building efforts in rural development described two decades ago by Paolo Freire in *Pedagogy of the oppressed* (Harmondsworth, Penguin, 1972), and of the early successes of primary health care in bringing about equity and self-reliance.

The challenge for those implementing home care and community involvement is to ensure the sustainability of these activities, particularly where resources are limited and demand for HIV/AIDS care is growing. Outreach from hospitals with specialized teams may be neither feasible nor cost-effective if each village has 10 or 20 homes with affected families. It would be interesting to see whether an existing primary health care programme or other community-based programme can sustain home care and community involvement efforts by restructuring health care priorities in line with assessed needs.

No ready-made solutions can be given for home care and community involvement. Communities and health care providers must develop their own models of home and community care according to local conditions and traditions.

CHAPTER 7

Developing management for primary health care

J.P. Ranken

During the 1980s it became clear that implementation of primary health care in many countries was being frustrated by lack of effective management. This was as true in Zambia as anywhere. The problem has been recognized, however, and in 1980 the "yellow book" *Health by the people: proposals for achieving health for all in Zambia* had set out an administrative structure for implementing and sustaining primary health care at community level. This was followed by a series of training workshops to help develop management skills among members of provincial and district teams so that they could take corporate responsibility for planning and implementation of primary health care programmes. Training manuals were produced on such topics as producing district plans, decision-making, developing team skills, implementing local programmes, costing, monitoring and evaluation.

By 1985, however, it was recognized that management skills—particularly as reflected in teamwork—were still poor among health personnel. A management development programme was introduced to tackle this problem, particularly at district level. New methods of training were developed at the same time as changes in management systems and organization.

Studying how district management teams work

In early 1985 the University of Zambia Department of Community Health and the Institute of Child Health, London, carried out a small study in the two Zambian districts of Mazabuka and Mumbwa. The purpose of the study was to examine how district management teams actually work in practice. The observations were made by medical students as part of their community health training. They sought to examine how members of district management teams related to each other, how accountability was pursued, how district priorities were established, how district management teams worked with other sectors and how the teams supported their local communities, including local community health workers. The study also observed the more conventional management activities of the district management teams with respect to planning, hospital management and transport. The study leaders subsequently discussed the findings with the teams concerned. The final report sought to combine the findings from the two districts with the findings of other evaluations available at the time, highlighting a number of important conclusions.

Progress was made in establishing primary health care through a network of rural health centres, community health committees and community health workers, and in providing support through primary health care coordinators and district management teams. The district teams produced plans for the future and developed systems to implement them. Some progress was made towards decentralization, with more effective decision-making at district level. Resources for management training were available in the Ministry of Health, the National Institute of Public Administration and the University of Zambia, though these were not always well coordinated.

A constantly reported problem was shortage of transport and poor management of what there was. A more fundamental problem, however, was the patchy commitment to primary health care. There were large gaps in the understanding of primary health care, especially in relation to community roles and potential and to opportunities for change in medical services. Roles within district management teams were not always clear. Leadership was variable, especially where there was no District Medical Officer, or where there was one who was not oriented to primary health care. District management teams had grown in size and were often unwieldy or ineffective. Information and financial control systems were weak and systems were needed for intersectoral collaboration and hospital decision-making. Provinces gave poor support to districts, and districts in turn failed to give enough support to rural health centres to enable them to work effectively with their local communities.

In the face of such problems the Ministry of Health, with Swedish assistance, was involved in a programme to strengthen health management and infrastructure. Projects were under way to improve supply and maintenance of transport, to extend and upgrade rural health centres, to strengthen planning, budgeting and information systems, and to provide management training. The major challenge for management development, however, was to introduce a programme that was economical to provide, straightforward to operate and capable of running within the existing health system.

A three-year management development programme

The report of the study of district management teams in Mazabuka and Mumbwa reinforced an already growing awareness that urgent action was needed to improve management of primary health care. Initial enthusiasm for primary health care had frequently given way to open disillusionment. Health workers had encountered operational problems which they were unable to solve alone. There seemed to be more rhetoric than reality in giving primary health care priority over secondary and tertiary medical care. Many influential people did not seem to appreciate what was involved in implementing primary health care. Above all, however, there were constraints resulting from a declining economy which led to cutbacks in public spending and reductions in living standards, not least for health workers in outlying areas.

Within the Ministry of Health itself, the main sources of development funds were external donors. With a few notable exceptions these donors tended to favour separately planned "vertical" programmes, many of which made use of training courses and workshops that were poorly coordinated, attended by the same people and gave insufficient attention to putting ideas into practice. In such a situation conventional management training was unlikely to be successful so a new system had to be devised. This emphasized learning within the work situation, strengthened and made use of management teams at each level, used current problems as the agenda for training and used managers themselves as key trainers. The training stressed the responsibility of managers for applying the results of training to their everyday work.

The programme focused on strengthening three management areas: planning, budgeting and financial control; information; and primary health care support.

Work was already under way in the Ministry of Health Planning Unit to improve planning, budgeting and financial control, which worked according to an annual cycle. It was planned to use this annual cycle as the framework for training provincial and district teams. Quarterly workshops for these teams would deal with the production of district forward plans and priorities, the translation of forward plans into estimates, the reconciliation of estimates with financial allocations, and control of expenditure in the light of actual allocations. Training inputs would be provided by the planning unit, and provincial teams would help district teams to prepare plans and monitor implementation.

In relation to management information, the emphasis was on helping districts to develop and maintain their own information systems as part of the national system. This entailed several steps: identifying the essential information required by district management teams for monitoring activities on a monthly basis, helping district managers to monitor activities through key indicators, and establishing local reporting systems at community, rural health centre and district levels prior to sending information to higher levels.

The existing primary health care support system was based on district management teams visiting rural health centres, and rural health centre teams visiting each community and community health worker at least monthly. In practice, this was rarely achieved because of various difficulties such as lack of transport. The new management development programme aimed to augment the monthly visits with a system of planned routine meetings. All community health workers would attend a meeting at their nearest rural health centre on a fixed day each month and, similarly, rural health centre staff would attend a monthly district workshop meeting. The intention was that at these meetings reports would be made, drugs and supplies issued, problems discussed and training given. The aim would be to use the meetings as team-building events that would maintain the motivation of peripheral health workers.

Setting up such a system, however, required firstly that district management teams give high priority to it and secondly that workers in rural health centres arrange to have regular contact with communities and community health workers. This would entail routine joint meetings and workshops for district management teams and regional health centre teams, as well as regular meetings for village representatives in each health centre area. The same system could be used for collecting and discussing information as part of the district's management information system. Finally, provincial management teams would have a key part to play in establishing and maintaining such a system by training and monitoring district management teams.

A three-year programme of "activity-based learning workshops" was therefore planned. This was intended to strengthen and integrate different management systems and provide a framework for improved communication throughout the entire Ministry of Health structure. It was hoped that, by establishing a routine pattern of workshops, the need for uncoordinated ad hoc courses and workshops would decrease. The final programme was based on regular workshops at four levels:

— national workshops for provincial teams (two a year, three days' duration);
— provincial workshops, run by each provincial management team for all district management teams in the province (quarterly, one or two days' duration);
— district workshops, run by each district management team for all rural health centre teams in the district (monthly, one day's duration);
— rural health centre workshops, run by each rural health centre team for all community health workers in the area (monthly, one day's duration).

Clear objectives were set for the workshops at each level of the health system.

One objective of the national workshops for provincial health teams was to ensure a common approach to primary health care throughout the country by implementing an integrated training and support system. Other objectives were to train provincial teams as trainers of district teams, to serve as a major channel of communication between Ministry of Health headquarters and the provinces, and to produce provincial action plans for strengthening management and primary health care support.

Objectives of the provincial workshops for district management teams were: to agree district plans and review their implementation; to discuss current problems in districts and work out solutions; to monitor implementation of the new systems of primary health care support, information, and planning, budgeting and financial control; and to train district management teams in management and the running of workshops for health centre teams.

Monthly meetings run by district management teams for health centre teams were intended to coordinate plans for health centres and communities and receive reports of health centre and community activities. In addition, the meetings could be used to distribute drugs, supplies and monthly salary cheques to health centre staff. Part of each meeting would consist of training related to current needs and problems. The meetings would end with agreement on action plans in order to ensure progress from one meeting to the next.

Similar aims were set for the monthly meetings between health centre staff and village representatives (community health workers and others) in their area, with distribution of drugs and supplies, reports on current activities, training related to local needs and problems, and action plans to summarize action to be taken before the next meeting.

The three-year programme started in February 1987 with a briefing of all provincial teams. Two headquarters/provincial workshops were held in the first year and a third took place in April 1988.

At these high-level workshops, a three-part pattern was established. The workshop began with a review of current problems and issues raised by both the headquarters and provincial teams. The central part of each workshop consisted of joint problem-solving, inputs of new information (such as on the budgeting system or recent developments in AIDS) and sessions on management skills (such as delegation and handling conflict). Each workshop ended with the preparation of action plans by the provincial team and the headquarters team, identifying action they would take before the next workshop. The action plans were a useful means of monitoring progress by teams at both provincial and headquarters level.

During the first year a major task of the workshops was to work with provincial management teams on the details of how they would run similar workshops for their own district teams. Towards the end of the year, the provincial teams began to have regular workshops with their districts, and during the second year some district teams started regular meetings with the teams from their own health centres.

A mid-term evaluation took place in the middle of the second year and highlighted a number of improvements. There was evidence of improved communication between provincial management teams and the headquarters planning unit. The provincial teams were becoming more skilled in problem-solving, dealing with staff, organizing workshops for district teams and improving such things as transport systems for supervisory visits. Provincial Medical Officers seemed to be getting a clearer idea of their managerial responsibilities and how to fulfil them.

In the districts, a number of improvements in management were noted. These included more regular and accurate reporting to provincial level and improved delegation, problem-solving, and transport allocation. Some districts made progress in integrating services for maternal and child health in clinics for children under five years of age, while others reported better control of health centre activities such as immunization coverage and inventory keeping.

The problems that remained in districts were those associated with transport shortages, intermittent drug supplies, irregular supervision of health centres, and coordination of centrally organized training courses. There was a feeling, however, that the regular pattern of workshops provided a means for district management teams to deal more positively with difficult problems.

Although there was some evidence of district management teams meeting more frequently with rural health centre teams, regular monthly contact proved difficult to sustain. This was unfortunate because it was at local level that frequent contact was most needed.

The district of Mazabuka provides an example of how a local system was developed. An informal meeting was arranged at the district head-quarters each month when health centre staff came to collect their monthly pay and supplies. These informal occasions were reinforced by more intensive residential workshops every four months in inexpensive school accommodation. In other districts workshops with health centre staff took place more intermittently but dealt with a wide range of issues, such as health centre security, outreach to local villages, implementation of im-munization programmes, collection and use of data, and general pro-gramme supervision.

Health centre staff felt the need to improve their own planning capabilities. There were also problems such as staff shortages and drugs control to be looked at in future workshops. A particular need was expressed for health centres to be supplied with books and training manuals to strengthen their own training work. This in turn highlighted the need for health centres to be involved in training and regular meetings with their own village representatives (community health workers, community lead-ers, etc.), which could be seen as the most crucial part of the whole management development exercise. Nevertheless, with the establishment of a communications system between all management levels, the stage was set for regular contacts between health centres and their surrounding com-munities to be strengthened.

Since the management development programme had improved management support for primary health care, it was decided to continue for a further three years. During this second period the programme continued to achieve its objectives of improving teamwork, communication and basic management skills at provincial and district levels. As in previous years, much more needed to be done at the level of rural health centres and villages. There was also a need to improve management at the Ministry of Health itself since it was responsible for the health system throughout the country.

The management development programme was strengthened by the addition of a component for training people as trainers in each province and district. Political change was imminent following the elections of 1991, so the need was increasingly seen for restructuring and change within the Ministry of Health. Many of the needed changes had been clearly identified through the management development programme.

There was an obvious need for the Ministry of Health to be clear about its own function of developing and maintaining a health system oriented to primary health care. This would entail a slimmed-down headquarters concerned with the strategic issues of policy development, resource allocation, personnel planning and initiation of change. With greater delegation of authority to provincial and other levels, the Ministry of Health role would be to ensure coordination and communication between the many different parts of the health system. The management development programme had produced a framework for coordination with regular joint meetings and workshops at each level; it was now for the Ministry of Health to ensure that the system worked, with clear procedures, targets and performance indicators agreed at each level.

The management development programme placed great emphasis on effective teamwork at each level. This was still needed, especially at the level of the rural health centre and local community. Teamwork would also help improve intersectoral cooperation. Another important task was to identify individual leaders at each level and hold them administratively accountable for developing and improving the effectiveness of their teams.

Training was needed to go hand in hand with improvements to management systems. There was the reintroduction of training for community health workers, training for health centre teams, and a continuing programme of management development for those, particularly doctors, in positions of managerial responsibility.

Nurse management support for primary health care

Nurses have played a predominant role in the development of primary health care in Zambia, as they have in many other countries. In the absence of a strong lead from doctors, nurses were quick to appreciate the importance of primary health care. There were already nurses throughout the country, particularly in rural areas. They were already considerably involved in preventive work in mother and baby clinics, in nutrition programmes and in health education. With the advent of primary health care, new nursing categories were created. Community health nurses were to work at grass-roots level, and a new postgraduate course in community health gave nurse graduates skills similar to those of a doctor qualified in public health.

Yet nurses remained in a position subservient to doctors. They had the skills and qualities for primary health care, but not the authority and control over resources to fulfil their leadership potential.

The part played by nurses in primary health care and the scope for strengthening their role in organization and management became clear during the initial studies of the work of district management teams. An opportunity to follow this up came in 1988 when the Ministry of Health responded to an invitation to take part in a more detailed study, funded by the United Kingdom Overseas Development Administration, of nursing management and primary health care in Africa.

Zambian nurses collected data by interviewing nurses and other staff at district and health centre levels in the Lusaka and Copperbelt Provinces. This gave an urban bias to the findings, which was inevitable because of transport difficulties at the time. It also highlighted the fact that health resources, including those of nursing personnel, were disproportionately concentrated in urban areas.

As indicated above, the nursing profession responded to the challenge of primary health care with the creation of a new category of community nurse. Family health nurses are community nurses based at health centres where they help provide primary health care services. They are active in areas such as maternal and child health and immunization and they support primary health care in local communities, in close cooperation with community health workers and traditional birth attendants.

There is a need for clarification of the nature of community-based primary health care. Many nurses believe their role is to provide services for communities, rather than to work with them and with other agencies to identify and tackle problems together. Where nurses are well versed in the processes of community development for health they are able to carry out community diagnosis, seek solutions to problems with the community, plan joint strategies to tackle the problems and support community efforts in implementing plans. The focal point for support of primary health care is the local health centre but this was frequently found to be isolated. Although nurses used their initiative to overcome local problems, they often felt constrained by a lack of support and encouragement from their own managers. Within health centres there were also sometimes unresolved conflicts between medical assistants and nurses which adversely affected leadership in the centre and the centre's own work in the community.

There was considerable potential for nurse managers to take a strong lead in primary health care. They had a large resource of nurses throughout the country, appropriate training schemes had been developed, nurses had good working relationships with other professions and, as a predominantly female profession, nurses identified easily with issues of women's health. Nurses had high professional standards of competence and reliability, they identified closely with communities and individuals, and they had the practical management skills that ward sisters and district public health nurses need.

Despite such positive factors, however, nurses had to contend with very real constraints. These included their initial hospital-based training, an over-reliance on foreign professional role models, the medical domination of nursing and a preponderance of nurses in urban areas, as well as limited authority in decision-making, controlling resources, prescribing medication and treating patients.

Implications for the future

This chapter has described various activities undertaken to improve management support for primary health care in Zambia. The range of activities illustrates how action is needed at many points in the country's health management system. The whole system needs to be kept under continuous review for there is no part of it that does not have a distinctive contribution to make in support of primary health care. The future of primary health care in Zambia is problematic at best. It will be assured only if a key phrase in the Declaration of Alma-Ata is taken seriously: "Primary health care . . . forms an integral part both of the country's health system, of which it is the central function and main focus, and of the overall social and economic development of the community."

There are many pressures to divert attention from primary health care as the "central function and main focus" of Zambia's health system. Many of these are severe economic pressures. Lack of foreign exchange for fuel and spare parts causes havoc in a system based on local, and often remote, communities. This leads to disillusionment, frustration and the breakdown of normal working in many places. In a situation of severe economic decline, attention to priorities is of paramount importance. It might be assumed that Zambia's priority would be to maintain primary health care as the basis of its health system, but there is much evidence that this is not the case. National statements about health needs are frequently expressed in terms of shortage of doctors and the need for more hospitals. It is as if earlier statements about the effectiveness of primary health care had never been made. This lack of commitment to primary health care is compounded by offers of funding for equipment, hospitals and doctors made by wealthy donor agencies.

Zambia is also caught up in the worldwide economic trend towards market-oriented capitalism and away from state provision of public services. Thus the whole notion of a nationwide health infrastructure firmly rooted in primary health care, which Zambia has struggled to build up over the past 10 years, is thrown into question. The trend is seen in the introduction of charges for health services and the establishment of the University Teaching Hospital in Lusaka as an independent concern. The role of NGOs is also assuming greater prominence, as they are seen to be relatively well managed and therefore more deserving of support from multilateral and bilateral aid agencies. Paradoxically, these influences are coming at a time when key positions in the Ministry of Health such as those of Provincial Medical Officer are becoming fully "Zambianized", and the occupants of those posts are gaining confidence and understanding of their role in a system of primary health care. At the same time nurses are gaining a clearer understanding of their role, and how they can give real leadership to primary health care in the field.

The way that other problems are faced will also be a major challenge for primary health care in Zambia. The impact of AIDS is horrific and shows no sign of diminishing. Yet community-based approaches, which build on an existing primary health care infrastructure such as that in Mazabuka, are proving effective and are receiving international recognition.

Decentralization, where it has been carried through in urban areas, has been shown to have major benefits. Some signs can be detected of a shift of people back to rural areas as a result of the poverty, unemployment and food shortages in towns, although the shift is by no means pronounced. Many of the educated elite are maintaining their rural links as a safeguard against urban decline and as possible havens for retirement. All this could lead to new life for rural areas if scope is given for rural initiatives and policies of decentralization are followed through.

On the political front, the growth of multiparty democracy may lead to changes similar to those now taking place in many parts of the world. In the past, health and community development in Zambia has entailed linking party structures to local decision-making processes, and this has been the foundation of primary health care in many local communities. This may change along with moves to strengthen market influences in more areas of health and social care.

Against all these changes the need for far-sighted, flexible and adaptable management will be crucial. Signs of this management style were apparent in Zambia's management development programme, not least in efforts made at the highest levels in the Ministry of Health to identify problems and work through them constructively and openly, and in the commitment of nurses to fulfil their leadership roles in primary health care. Such approaches to management will be crucial during the 1990s if the advances made in primary health care during the 1980s are to be continued.

CHAPTER 8

Monitoring and evaluation of primary health care

P.J. Freund & K. Kalumba

This chapter describes the results of a longitudinal community-based study sponsored by the United Nations Children's Fund (UNICEF) and commissioned by the interministerial committee of the Government of Zambia and UNICEF. The general purpose of the study, which began in 1982, was to investigate problems in providing health services to remote rural populations and to evaluate and monitor the impact of primary health care. Because the research focused on impact measures and was action-oriented, the results were of direct concern to the Ministry of Health's efforts to promote primary health care as national policy.

The study looked at the health status of a sample of families in selected rural communities with special attention to women and children. It was decided to monitor the health of selected households over a four-year period. The research was also intended to monitor availability and utilization of various components of the primary health care programme in order to assess impact and identify constraints to effective implementation. Researchers monitored community health planning, including the consultative process by which each community chose its community health worker. A documentation of the process would explain how people in communities with few economic resources and with limited formal education could be motivated to take more responsibility for preventive health measures. The researchers hoped to find out how community participation could be implemented and sustained.

Another important overall component of the project was to provide information to the Government of Zambia and UNICEF on specific areas of need in relation to health workers and the village communities and to offer suggestions for improvements in health care delivery. The research team became involved in facilitating improvements in health care delivery once problems were identified (such as requesting equipment from UNICEF to maintain the vaccine cold chain and setting up better health recording systems).

The information gathered was intended to benefit both the communities concerned and the Ministry of Health's Department of Maternal and Child Health. The data were also presented on a regular basis to the joint Government/UNICEF committee and were used by UNICEF in formulating the joint programme of operations.

The setting

Fieldwork began in January 1982 and continued until July 1986. Two remote rural areas were selected in Western and Northern Provinces. In both places primary health care was in its early stages (i.e. training of community health workers). The two areas were sufficiently different in terms of environment so that comparisons and contrasts could be made. The Luampungu research site in Sesheke District of Western Province has about 1600 inhabitants in 18 villages scattered along the three main rivers. The population density is two per square kilometre and the area can be described as semi-desert.

The villagers are mainly subsistence farmers. There is a notable lack of cash crops and few available outlets for marketing them. Moreover, there are few retail outlets in which to purchase goods. The average per capita income at the time was 50 Zambian kwacha a year (equivalent to about US$50 in 1982). There is one school in the ward, located in Luampungu compound, with 210 students in grades 1–7.

Kabinga study site is located in Mpika District of Northern Province and has a population of 3150 people in 17 villages along the shores of Lake Chaya. The people live mainly from fishing but also cultivate cassava in the relatively infertile swampland. Their diet is supplemented by subsidiary crops and most villages have small plots for fruit.

Heavy rainfall makes the area inaccessible during the rainy season (December–April). Some villages are also inaccessible by vehicle even during the dry season and transport is by canoe. The area is served by two primary schools (grades 1–7), a small grocery store, a government rural health centre and a mobile market. There is an active trade network involving fish, maize meal, bread, sugar, soap and other goods. As a result of fishing, the average per capita income in Kabinga was 350 Zambian kwacha a year.

Methodology and sampling

Health should be seen as more than an individual's search for care. Rather, it is a community's concern and ability to maintain health. This necessitates a broader view which takes into account the social system, the environment, and the political and economic system, and how these affect the individual's ecosystem or the community's health status. The study aimed not only at isolating factors related to individual sociodemographics and health-seeking behaviour, but also at monitoring community changes that might have an impact on health status (such as agricultural schemes, significant out-migration, community participation in health promotion, literacy programmes, and so on). Information was gathered from formal and informal discussions with a wide range of local community and district administration leaders as well as household surveys and available records.

The household survey instrument consisted of items on illness, mortality, nutrition, maternal and reproductive history, and utilization of health services by the household with particular emphasis on women and children. The data gathering was designed to answer the following questions:

- What specific socioeconomic and demographic variables are related to health status or health-seeking behaviour of household members in this community?
- What is the status of health/nutrition in this community?
- What is the level of use of various health services by this community and what factors, internal and external, affect that use?
- To what extent are community members involved in participative health care and to what extent are auxiliary staff, such as community health workers and traditional healers, effectively accepted and utilized?
- What major constraints affect the implementation of community-based health care?
- What evidence exists of intersectoral cooperation?

To answer these questions it was necessary to select key indicators of major variables such as socioeconomic condition, health status, health service utilization, nutrition level, and sanitation and water supply. In addition to data collection, the fieldwork focused on improving methods, defining variables and refining techniques. Luampungu and Kabinga were visited at approximately three-month intervals with two weeks spent in each area; additional trips were made to other areas to provide comparisons. In total seven months were spent in the field over the four-year period.

After the pilot survey and a comparative baseline study, it was decided to use 100 households that would form the core sample to be monitored over the next four years.

The sampling frame was all villages within Luampungu Ward and the Kabinga rural health centre catchment area in which there was a family of childbearing age (i.e. where the youngest child was below five years and/or the woman was still below age 45). A simple random selection process was used to obtain a sample of 100 households (approximately eight per village).

Major findings

Disease patterns

Disease patterns were determined both by retrospective recall and data collected prospectively. Questions relating to health variables concerned the respondents' assessment of episodes of illness in members of the household, health-seeking behaviour, and attitudes towards health and nutrition. The most common diseases reported by households within the previous three months in both Luampungu and Kabinga were diarrhoea, upper respiratory infections, malaria, hepatitis and malnutrition. However, the distribution of these diseases differed between the two areas and seemed to reflect the contrasting environments. Malaria and upper respiratory infections were more common in Kabinga than in Luampungu. On the other hand, hepatitis and chronic malnutrition were more common in Luampungu, which reflects the poor housing, poor sanitation, continuing drought and inadequate food supply in the area.

The distribution of the most common illnesses conforms to the pattern seen at the rural health centres, mission hospital and district hospitals, and is similar to that in other parts of Zambia, except for the relatively high incidence of hepatitis. It should be stressed, however, that these illnesses reflect national health categories and obscure many of the community's real health concerns. For instance, the prospectively collected household health data revealed a high incidence of headache, as well as "folk diseases" such as *singumbe* in Luampungu. These were obviously a major concern but were not reflected in national statistics or health centre records. The symptoms of *singumbe* are described as firstly a headache and stiff neck, progressing rapidly to ulcerations of the anus and eventual death in 3–4 days if left untreated. It was commonly believed that the only effective treatment was medicine from a traditional healer, so few cases were brought to the rural health centres or mission hospital.

Many of the most common diseases are clearly related to the environment and can be addressed by primary health care through improved sanitation, health education and advice on agriculture and nutrition. Several meetings were held with local leaders and community health workers to discuss the role of the community in reducing disease by improving sanitation, boiling water and digging pit latrines.

Nutrition

A major part of the study was an attempt to find a way of assessing the nutritional status of the community, and especially its children. The general assumption was that the conditions of children would be indicative of the state of health of the community. The nutritional survey showed that 27% of the children measured in Luampungu and 16% in Kabinga fell below the 13.5 cm standard for upper arm circumference during the initial survey. This reflects poor nutrition in Luampungu when compared with Kabinga. The problems of Luampungu villagers have been exacerbated by periods of drought, lack of agricultural advice and an inadequate infrastructure.

There was a clear deterioration of general nutritional status in both areas during the four years of the study. In Luampungu this was caused by low production levels, out-migration of young males and drought. In Kabinga a contributing factor was the rural–urban trade imbalance which led to more and more fish being marketed to purchase essential commodities. District agricultural extension officers have been encouraged to advise on the efficient use of fertilizer, drought-resistant crops and better production techniques in Luampungu. In Kabinga the problem is less easy to solve as more and more fishermen are becoming involved in the cash trade and stocks of fish are decreasing in Lake Chaya.

Interventions designed to reduce malnutrition should be focused on the children aged under 2 years who are at risk. Preventive activities should include promotion of oral rehydration therapy, promotion of breast-feeding, immunizations, nutrition, education, promotion of balanced food production, and the treatment and prevention of diseases such as malaria, acute respiratory illness, worms and anaemia.

Maternal and reproductive data

Complete reproductive histories were collected from 111 mothers in Luampungu and 101 in Kabinga (including all wives in polygamous households).

The mean age at first marriage and at first pregnancy is lower in Kabinga and reflects a still common cultural practice of child betrothal in that area. The markedly higher percentage of difficulties in childbirth in Luampungu (33%) tended to occur in women who had a history of stillbirths and miscarriages. Reported childbirth difficulties among Kabinga women (8%) were concentrated in those aged 15–17 (a defined risk group).

Total pregnancies in Luampungu were 609, with 420 in Kabinga. Miscarriages (6%) and stillbirths (5%) resulted in a higher pregnancy wastage rate in Luampungu (12%) than in Kabinga (7%). The under-five mortality rate was also higher in Luampungu. The majority of women gave birth at home (78% in Luampungu and 90% in Kabinga) and a substantial number were assisted by a traditional birth attendant (27% in Luampungu, 16% in Kabinga). Most women were attended by a close relative (41% in Luampungu, 56% in Kabinga). Twelve per cent of women in both areas gave birth alone. Accessibility of a hospital or clinic is an important factor: in Kabinga the district hospital at Mpika (100 km distant) is the nearest facility that can handle deliveries.

The high risk for mothers in Luampungu points to the importance of training traditional birth attendants, particularly for screening "at-risk" women, for encouraging tetanus immunization and for providing health education. In Kabinga, the presence of a trained midwife at the rural health centre would have encouraged more mothers to attend antenatal clinics because many had refused to be seen by a male medical assistant.

Health service utilization

Studies in East Africa have shown a close correlation between the proximity of health services and their use. In Uganda the average number of outpatient visits declines by 60% for every two miles (3.2 km) that people live from a hospital, and every one and a half miles (2.4 km) from a dispensary. In Zambia, 21% of the population live more than 12 km from a health centre. Distance was clearly an important factor in utilization of health services in Luampungu and Kabinga.

Responses to the question "What action is taken when the child becomes ill?" showed a high proportion of self-care (39% in Luampungu, 22% in Kabinga) and use of traditional healers (19% in Luampungu, 16% in Kabinga). This is probably related to the long distance to the health centre, particularly in Luampungu where the distance to the nearest rural health centre (Nawinda) is 44 km. The sandy soil and hot climate also hinder travel. Patients must walk or be taken by ox-drawn sledge for two days to reach the health centre. Moreover, because of the frequent lack of drugs or absence of personnel, patients delay going to the health centre and often bypass it for the mission hospital where drugs are available (75 km distant). Most mothers in Luampungu said they waited an average of 2.5 days before going to the clinic and in some cases would wait for as long as seven days. Access is less problematic in Kabinga because most villages lie within a few hours walk of the rural health centre. However, drugs are frequently in short supply and patients often travel instead to the mission clinic (5–6 hours' walking distance) to obtain them. During the rainy season most of the villages in Kabinga are cut off from the health facilities and drug deliveries to the under-five clinics are disrupted. Although a substantial proportion (64% in Luampungu, 72% in Kabinga) used the clinics regularly, a considerable number of mothers (24% in Luampungu, 21% in Kabinga) said they did not attend.

In areas like Luampungu an effective community health worker is vital. The fact that a health centre is geographically accessible does not necessarily mean there is effective access in terms of drugs and services. Because of the general shortage of drugs in Zambia many health centres often have few drugs and consequently cannot supply the needs of the growing number of community health workers. There are currently plans by the Ministry of Health to establish rural health centres in Luampungu when funds become available. Moreover, additional community health workers will be trained in both areas. In order for community health workers to function effectively, however, they must have supervision, transport (i.e. bicycles), drugs and equipment.

Health recording

A serious obstacle to accurate understanding of the patterns of health service utilization and their effects on the health of the community is the lack of a reliable information system. A possible solution to current problems of inadequate and sometimes unreliable health data generated by routine recording in rural health centres could be to explore and test alternative methods of collecting data. One method that has been tried involves the use of schoolchildren to collect data from their villages. Thirteen of the 18 villages in Luampungu are represented in the school and all of the Kabinga villages are represented in the two primary schools in the area. Teachers were requested to ask pupils each week about births, deaths and major illnesses in their villages. Follow-up showed that this exercise not only provided useful data but generated interest in health matters among students and villagers. It also served as a useful way of informing the community health worker of problems needing attention. Such a system can be important for recording births and deaths, since village registers are rarely kept up to date.

A village household recording system has been introduced and will provide baseline data on illnesses which should facilitate future evaluation. Survey cards were distributed to a sample of 50 households in each area. The recorder, either the head of household or a schoolchild, marked down each time someone in the household suffered from complaints such as headache, backache, fever, abdominal pains and injuries. The type of treatment sought (clinic, traditional herbs/healer), or no treatment, was also recorded. Because of the high rate of return, the recording system was expanded to all 100 households in each study site as well as 50 additional households selected at random.

The survey card was designed to be used also for clinic visits. The rural health centres, the mission hospital's mobile services and the community health workers were informed about the purpose of the survey card. These service providers were given a list of the 100 households and advised to monitor them.

The rural health centres were given a register for recording all visits from members of the sample households as well as other data (i.e. drug supplies, equipment, transport, outbreaks of disease). This register serves to monitor the use of health services.

The success of these community data collection systems shows the potential of such methods for generating information that is of immediate practical use to the community, the community health worker, the village health committee and rural health centre staff. There is often a tendency to emphasize the importance of data compiled at national level and distributed to the districts and communities rather than focusing on giving the rural health centre staff and community health workers the skills to collect data which they can use. Even if aggregate data could be disseminated rapidly to rural health centres, it is often in a form that has little relevance to a particular area. It is therefore more reasonable to concentrate efforts on training community health workers, health assistants, traditional birth attendants and clinical officers in simple techniques of data collection and analysis. Efforts in this direction are now under way as part of ongoing training programmes.

Implementation of primary health care

One of the major objectives of the study was to monitor the implementation of primary health care, to identify problems that might hinder the process and to suggest improvements. The study showed the importance of politics in primary health care, from national level down to community level. During the first visit to Luampungu it became clear that the researchers were being used by the ward councillor to convince the community that food relief, and ultimately a rural health centre, would be brought to the area. In Kabinga the local chief viewed primary health care as a way to collect revenue. In addition, village rivalries arose over who should be trained as community health workers and where they should reside. The collection, storage and allocation of drugs in Luampungu became a hotly contested issue involving the school headmaster, the village health committee, the village headmen and the ward councillor.

The issue is not whether primary health care is political or non-political, because achieving health for all cannot be anything but political. Social development is an inherently political process. Because primary health care implies a sharing of power, local political interests will often perceive new power-holders as a threat. In some areas, power is regarded as both constant and limited, and if new power-holders arise they are not easily accommodated within the existing sociopolitical structure. In Zambia, problems arose because of a misunderstanding of the process of primary health care and the role of local politicians in that process. There were also other issues that were evident in the study areas, as well as in many areas of Zambia. For example, the selection of a young community health worker who begins to challenge older traditional authority sets modernity against tradition. The role of women may become an issue if women are chosen as community health workers or given an active role on village health committees when traditionally only men made decisions. Conflicts may develop over tribal issues when different groups reside in the same area. There are also political issues regarding the distribution of resources, decentralization and government directives on when and how primary health care should be implemented.

Experience in Luampungu and Kabinga has shown how important it is to educate district and local politicians about primary health care and involve them in it. This means that the first step should be the formation of a district health management team that is intersectoral and involves ward councillors. One of the functions of this group is to educate those involved about the meaning of primary health care, its relationship to social development and the roles that ward councillors, teachers and health workers can play in the process. A village health committee should then be formed to play a similar role in relation to local issues. The village committee should also discuss the selection of community health workers. It has often been the case that the first step in implementing primary health care has been to tell communities to select community health workers according to guidelines from the Ministry of Health. As a result ward councillors usually selected relatives or other persons independently, without consulting their constituents or a village health committee. The persons chosen were in many cases inappropriate. The issue is clearly the devolution of power from the centre to the district and the community. Even if proper procedures are followed and the district politicians and local leaders are involved, it is still difficult to convince local communities to make the decision when the directive comes from the government. This has consequences later when communities ask the government to pay the community health workers because the government wanted them. These issues require constant education about primary health care at all levels. This means frequent discussions not only with politicians and health personnel but also with responsible persons from other sectors such as agriculture, education and sanitation.

District medical officers, mission health personnel and rural health centre staff have often noted that primary health care cannot succeed as long as curative care remains erratic. Clearly, there must be a balance between curative and preventive care. Community health workers who cannot provide drugs like aspirin and chloroquine will have little success in persuading villagers to dig latrines and rubbish pits and engage in preventive activities. It is therefore vital that every effort should be made to support rural health centres and community health workers with the drugs and equipment they need in order to work effectively.

Community participation: expectations

Community involvement is a major component of primary health care implementation and it was a major focus of the study. During the initial visit to Luampungu it became obvious that what the community expected was a rural health centre and they saw the researchers as the people who would provide it. The community was reinforced in this view by the ward councillor who wanted to satisfy community demands for his own political advantage. This became a constant source of tension throughout the project and required repeated explanations of what the researchers could and could not do. The villages of Luampungu had already experienced a series of disappointments. They built a self-help clinic but no one was available to staff it, they had been promised agricultural extension advice which never materialized, and they had grown cash crops that were never marketed because of the poorly developed infrastructure. A sociomedical survey for a schisto-somiasis project was associated by the villagers with the death of several children from measles soon after the researchers had left. As a result the villagers were both resistant to and suspicious of yet another survey which simply asked questions and gave them nothing in return. A community's expectations and previous experience with development projects are important factors to consider in the implementation of primary health care. In some countries, villagers offered the option of primary health care have turned it down. In most cases, once they see the improvements in the villages that have accepted it, they change their minds. Villages are not homogeneous and they should not be regarded as such.

Measuring impact

When the community-based study ended in 1986 sufficient baseline and monitoring information had been collected to permit an evaluation of the impact of child health and nutrition services in the two research areas. Although four years is too short a time to measure medical impact on morbidity and infant mortality, it is possible to see some changes and some social impact.

While this was not an intervention study, there have been a number of observable changes. Some can be attributed to project activities and some have resulted from the implementation of primary health care. There has been a significant rise in general awareness of health problems and preventive strategies in both study areas. The mere fact that households were involved in keeping a record of their illnesses resulted in more awareness of health. Members of these households started to raise questions about their health problems and how to alleviate them. In Kabinga a major change occurred when Chief Kabinga worked with the health assistant to improve sanitation in the area by building rubbish pits, latrines and permanent houses. The data collection process which aimed to link the schools, the community health worker and the community also made the community more aware of health issues and how they could be dealt with. The use of schoolchildren as health promoters seems to have great potential, especially in isolated rural communities, provided that teachers are trained in basic health issues, are given appropriate materials and involve the community health worker or rural health centre in the process.

The presence of a community health worker in the communities has made a significant impact. This is especially the case in Luampungu where the nearest rural health centre is a long distance away. If community health workers are given sufficient drugs, dressings and other medical supplies they can deal with more than 80% of the health problems in the community. They can also ensure that persons at risk or in need of urgent care are referred to the hospital or health centre. Community health workers can also work closely with health assistants in promoting preventive activities for health (such as pit latrines, nutrition education, oral rehydration, sanitation and general hygiene).

Despite changes in awareness and improvements in some general health practices, it cannot be denied that the overall situation has remained fairly static and even deteriorated over the years. The communities have been hampered by drought, a worsening of rural–urban trade, and the effects of general economic decline in Zambia. This has been reflected in a steadily falling level of nutrition in children and a sense of hopelessness in the communities. People see their position now as worse than it was 10 years ago.

Any evaluation, no matter how well designed, is useful only if the results are channelled to appropriate policy-makers. Researchers also have an obligation to inform the community of the results so that changes can be effected. This was done through meetings with local leaders, teachers and the community health workers. Research findings and recommendations were discussed openly with villagers from Luampungu and Kabinga as well as with the district primary health care coordinator, the community health workers, ward councillors, village headmen and rural health centre staff. The meetings have enabled the community to understand more clearly what primary health care involves. There were also opportunities to sort out problems between different individuals and groups. The inherent difficulty in this type of meeting or discussion is that the researchers were often seen as representatives of the central government with the power to provide a rural health centre, build roads, bring food relief and revise price structures. It was therefore necessary for community meetings to be organized and chaired by the ward councillor or his representative. An attempt was made to ensure that the meetings were not concerned solely with health issues but with general development of which health is an important part. The research results were regularly communicated to district officials, the primary health care coordinator and hospital staff.

At national level, reports are circulated to relevant persons at the Ministry of Health, the National Food and Nutrition Commission, the National Primary Health Care Development Committee, the National Commission for Development Planning, the Ministry of Agriculture Planning Unit and the interministerial committee of the government and UNICEF. The researchers were members of the National Primary Health Care Development Committee and presented detailed reports for discussion and action by relevant government officials. In December 1985 a major evaluation workshop was held. This brought together people doing monitoring and evaluation studies in agriculture, the nutrition industry, and education and provided an opportunity to share experiences from a variety of perspectives. The workshop was followed by a book which will serve as a guide[1] for further monitoring and evaluation studies in Zambia.

Finally, results were shared with other researchers and health workers through seminars and articles published in academic journals. Articles published in *Bwino*, which is circulated to all health personnel in Zambia, were well received and a large number of clinical officers and health assistants wrote asking for more information on the study. Governmental and nongovernmental organizations are expected to use the data in planning health service programmes.

Conclusion

Most previous monitoring and evaluation studies of health status have relied on output measures for evaluation (e.g. number of health clinics, outpatient attendances, and so on) instead of impact measures (such as the health status over time of women and children in the clinic area). The research goal of this study was to monitor the process of community participation in health care, to evaluate the delivery of health and nutrition services and to assess their impact in two rural communities over a four-year period. In view of Zambia's commitment to primary health care, it is important to provide data from community-based research on the effectiveness of present institutional frameworks and the problems that may arise in shifting towards community responsibility for health.

While this study took a different approach to evaluating primary health care than that taken by other reviews and evaluations, all identified similar constraints and problems, such as lack of supervision, unreliable record systems, lack of community support for community

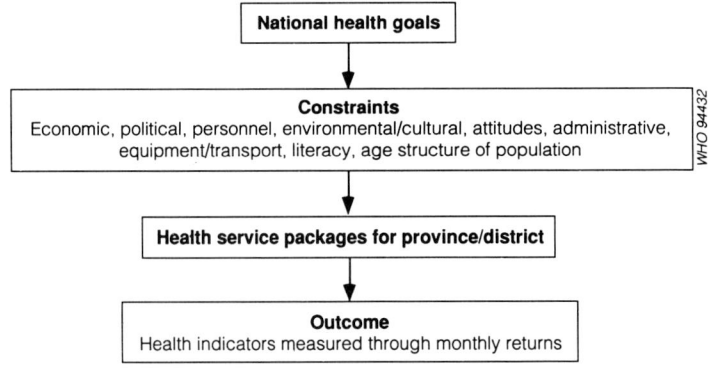

Fig. 1 National goals model

---

[1] Clarke R, Freund P. *Guidelines on project evaluation in Zambia*. Lusaka, University of Zambia, 1985.

health workers, inadequate transport and infrastructure, and shortages of personnel. These problems must be viewed against a background of rapid population growth, widespread poverty, deteriorating economic conditions and low levels of literacy. The current approach to health care delivery begins with national goals, mediated and filtered through constraints which lead to the delivery of health service "packages" to districts and provinces (see Fig. 1). The outcome is measured by various indicators (such as monthly returns from health centres and hospitals). These indicators, according to this model, provide a measure of health status and a sense of achievement of national health goals.

A more realistic approach with implications for national health planning and for implementation of primary health care conceives of the process as beginning from community needs and problems. These are in turn filtered through constraints and tackled using an integrated health care approach for the attainment of health goals (Fig. 2). The outcomes are measured by the degree to which health problems (such as child mortality and malnutrition) are reduced in the community.

The community-based approach assumes there is a need for knowledge of a particular community's health problems and needs. In some cases this knowledge may be acquired through survey research. In most instances, however, rural health centres, health workers, community health workers and local village leaders can provide the information.

Moreover, this framework has important implications for community perceptions of health problems and disease causation which will require more extensive health education. A continuing dialogue will be necessary between health workers, communities and planners. The emphasis on the community brings into sharper focus the normally silent and often neglected partner in the dialogue.

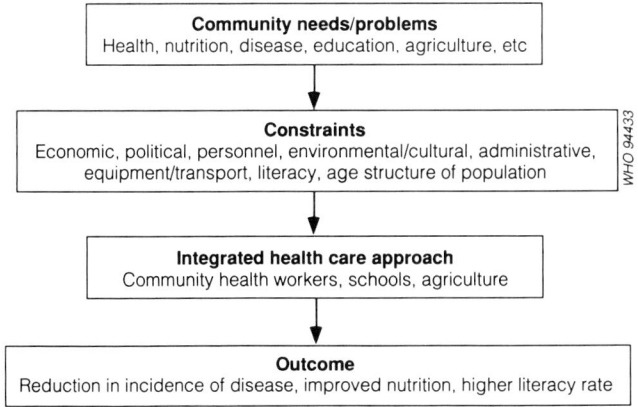

Fig. 2 Community-based model

Despite a great deal of health care planning in Zambia, indicators point to an urban bias and continued neglect of rural health care needs. Clearly rural areas like Luampungu and Kabinga pay a high price in disease morbidity resulting from the combined effects of drought, low agricultural production, poor water, poor sanitation, inaccessible health services, lack of political power and little infrastructure. At the same time significant changes and improvements can be made through effective implementation of primary health care supported by community participation and intersectoral cooperation.

CHAPTER 9

The role of traditional healers in primary health care in Zambia

P.A. Twumasi

Introduction

This report is based on a study carried out at the Institute for African Studies of the University of Zambia during 1983–84. The study sought to determine the status of traditional medicine in Zambia within the framework of a modern health care system.

The significance of the study derives from the thesis that traditional healers may have an important role to play in primary health care. Traditional healing is constantly adjusting to change. Structural and non-structural changes have emerged in the practice of traditional medicine and healers are seeking cooperation with the national health care delivery system. Such a cooperative effort will help to strengthen national health care.

Traditional healing institutions in Lusaka, Eastern and Luapula Provinces of Zambia were studied and traditional healers of different types were interviewed. Interviews were also conducted with members of the Traditional Healers Practitioners Association of Zambia (THPAZ), opinion leaders in provincial communities and clients of traditional healers. It was also deemed necessary to interview Ministry of Health officials as well as doctors and nurses at the University of Zambia Teaching Hospital in Lusaka.

Through the use of a questionnaire, interviews and panel discussion, field data were collected and analysed. Total respondents numbered 657, of which 222 were traditional healers, 300 clients of traditional healers, 79 opinion leaders and 56 doctors and nurses in the modern health system.

The changing role of traditional healers

A traditional healer or *Ng'anga* is a person with a recognized function in the community to deal with health and illness. He or she uses vegetable, animal and mineral substances and methods based on sociocultural traditions to deal with illness and to improve health. A traditional healer is recognized in the community as having competence to treat both relatives and non-relatives according to traditional practices. The healer heals in a recognized area and has a recognized clinic for consultation. People who occasionally treat or advise their own household members on health or illness are not included in this definition.

One notable feature of traditional healers is their concern to heal not just physical sickness but also psychological problems and even discord within a family or community. The instruction to live in harmony with relatives and neighbours was a common element of the advice given by traditional healers, according to the survey of their patients. It reflects the historical role of the village healer who not only was concerned with divination and the treatment of ills but also performed rituals to restore social harmony.

This combined role of traditional physician, psychiatrist and social worker gives the traditional healer a key role in preserving body, mind and community. In rural areas in the 1980s traditional healers were the first line of treatment for ailments—or, perhaps, concerns—of a social or psychological nature. Traditional healers themselves often classify diseases into those that occur naturally and those that have spiritual causes.

In Zambia, as elsewhere south of the Sahara before colonial contact, traditional medicine was the only medical service available to the sick. In the late 19th century, however, Zambia was colonized by Britain and as part of British institution-building a different type of medicine was introduced. The introduction of modern medicine (or what is sometimes referred to as Western medicine) was accompanied by official disapproval and discouragement of traditional medicine, which was accorded low status.

After independence in 1964 the Zambian Government encouraged the development and growth of indigenous institutions. It was within this frame of reference that traditional medicine also received encouragement.

A Witchcraft Act passed by the colonial authorities in 1914, with disastrous effects on traditional medicine, was amended in 1967. The amended act made it illegal for traditional healers to practise witchcraft but did not make other healing practices illegal so long as they were devoid of witchcraft. The act was seen as an attempt by the Government of Zambia to bring the practice of traditional medicine more into line with modern standards.

There were several very practical reasons for moving towards a more formal standardization of traditional medicine. There was, of course, the need to protect the clients of traditional healers from unsafe practices and to ensure the maintenance of certain accepted levels of practice. Traditional healers had never been required to possess specific qualifications or acquire authentication. Secondly there was the need to protect the healers themselves from persons who might bring their "profession" into disrepute through incompetence or unscrupulous behaviour. The later formation of an official National Association of

Traditional Healers came partly in response to this need. Lastly there was a need to regulate the fees paid to the healers.

Traditional medicine and the primary health care programme

At the initiative of the Ministry of Health and with the support of WHO and UNICEF, traditional healers and modern health practitioners met at a workshop in Lusaka in May 1977 to discuss traditional medicine and to outline the role of traditional healers in the development of primary health care in Zambia.

Workshop participants recommended that a National Association of Traditional Healers be formed to regulate the practice of traditional medicine. It was also recommended that a National Council of Traditional Healers be formed, by Act of Parliament and with government financing, in order to direct the affairs of traditional healers. While the association was later created, the council has not yet come into being.

Following the workshop, the Zambian Ministry of Health, in line with government policy, created an office for traditional medicine manned by a Schedule Officer. The principal duty of the Schedule Officer was to work in the area of traditional medicine and to help traditional healers improve their services through registration, refresher courses and standardization procedures. To this end the registration of traditional healers was put in motion. Traditional healers were asked, through their association's leaders, to seek help from the Schedule Officer at the Ministry of Health in order to improve their services. This and other moves increased available information on traditional medicine.

The acknowledgment that traditional healers have a role to play in medicine was an important step forward. Their role in society is indeed significant, if only because of the large numbers of people who consult them. During the colonial period, because of fear of disapproval, people coming to a physician or hospital would omit to mention, or even deny, that they had consulted a traditional healer first. In some cases presentation at a clinic might have been preceded by several months of treatment by a traditional healer, yet the patient would claim still to be in the early stages of the illness and to have taken no prophylactic measures. The open recognition of traditional healers by the authorities means that patients no longer hide the fact that they have tried traditional medicine first.

Types of traditional healer

There are four main types of traditional healer in Zambia: traditional birth attendants (traditional midwives), faith healers, spiritual healers (and diviners) and herbalists.

Traditional birth attendants

Traditional birth attendants (TBAs) focus their attention on pregnancy and assist women at childbirth. They are the midwives on whom rests the responsibility for delivering the child and caring for the health of the mother. They specialize in obstetrics but their activities extend to sex education and contraceptive counselling.

Most TBAs are middle-aged or elderly women. Most are illiterate or have little formal education. To them midwifery practice is a part-time occupation. It is estimated that about 80% of deliveries in rural areas are attended by traditional birth attendants.

TBAs learn their skills from relatives, through observation and apprenticeship. The trainee learns in an informal atmosphere while performing other household duties. Over a period of perhaps five years or more the apprentice picks up the skills and knowledge of TBA practice. She is trained in the preparation and administration of herbs needed for assisting deliveries, and she also learns how to remove the placenta and how to cut and dress the umbilical cord.

Patients who seek the services of TBAs are usually members of the same community. Thus TBAs tend to have an intimate knowledge of their patients. When a TBA is consulted by a pregnant woman, she carries out a physical examination to find out when delivery is due. She checks whether the baby is in the correct position. If all is well with the mother the TBA will ask the patient's relatives to prepare a place in their home for delivery to take place. For delivery, the mother is washed and put in a squatting position on the edge of a bed.

In addition to the TBA, one or two elderly women are usually present at delivery. When the baby is born and has cried, the placenta is removed and the umbilical cord is cut with a sharp instrument or with a special stone used for that purpose. Both baby and mother are washed with soap and water and the mother is asked to rest.

In difficult deliveries, the TBA's specialized knowledge as traditional healer is used. The TBA uses various herbal preparations for massage or to make drinks for the expectant mother in the hope of aiding delivery. When the problem is beyond the TBA's skill and there is a hospital or a clinic within reach, the expectant mother is usually taken to see a modern health practitioner for assistance. If no modern health service is available, the TBA must simply do what she can.

At the time of the study, Zambia had an ongoing training programme to upgrade the services of TBAs. More than 600 TBAs had been given refresher courses. In Mwachisompola, in Central Province, there was a combined programme for training community health workers and for giving refresher courses to TBAs. Mission and government hospitals and clinics were involved in the training programme.

Faith healers

Faith healers are often leaders of revivalist sects and African-based churches which have mushroomed in the country since independence. In addition to church services, leaders of these churches hold healing sessions. Some have clinics where patients (both churchgoers and non-churchgoers) go to seek help.

Faith healers use the Bible and prayer sessions to help "cure" patients who come to them. Certain days of the week may be set aside for healing. The faith healers are of both sexes, though most are male, and they deal with both social and psychological problems.

One of the faith healers interviewed during the course of this research was leader of a popular church called the Mutumwa Nchimi Church. He had many followers and the church had branches in Southern, Western and Eastern Provinces. Patients came from throughout the country for healing. Many were church members but a considerable number were not. The leader was known to have spiritual powers to heal epilepsy, sterility, impotence and asthmatic diseases. The faith healer had a healing clinic attached to the church building. Apart from treating outpatient cases he also had inpatients, especially those suffering from epilepsy. At the time of the research there were seven inpatients, aged between 14 and 19 years. It was difficult to distinguish between diagnostic and treatment procedures.

In one case a mother brought a boy of 15 years of age to the healer. The healer listened attentively to the mother and to her two sisters who had also come along. The mother gave the medical and social history of the child from birth up to the present. Without questioning, the faith healer took the mother and her child, who reportedly had suffered from fits, to an adjacent room. With the help of lighted candles and strongly scented perfume sprayed around the clinic, the faith healer offered prayers for the mother and child. He gave the child a ritual mark (with a white powder) on his forehead and on the top of his head. The mother and child were asked to report again in a week's time.

Before the treatment session the faith healer listened carefully to the patient's life story which had relevance to the patient's illness. He also had a discussion with the patient's relatives and they were asked to go back to their homes and live in harmony with each other and with the other members of their community. A month later, when the healer was visited again, the boy's mother confirmed that her son had had no more fits.

Spiritualists

Spiritualists, or diviners, use methods of possession, divination and other ritual means to diagnose illnesses and heal people. They claim to be intermediaries between the spirits and the patients who seek their help. They claim that their powers of healing and their diagnostic techniques come from spirits.

Spiritualists diagnose mainly through divination but when a spiritualist is satisfied that he has discovered what is wrong with a patient he often resorts to an interviewing technique to get more information to confirm the diagnosis. The spiritualist often seeks social and psychological reasons why an illness has occurred. He enquires about social disturbances, relationships that are upset, or inability on the part of the patient to communicate effectively with a relative in the household. The spiritualist will also ask about physical symptoms such as lack of appetite or inability to sleep.

All types of patient visit spiritualists. Usually these are patients who have failed to receive appropriate treatment from a modern health facility. Others feel that modern medical treatment would not be effective against their ills.

The problems usually dealt with by spiritualists are impotence, epilepsy, overweight, high blood pressure, unemployment, marital affairs, sexual problems and difficulties with partners, rheumatism, mental diseases, delirium, forgetfulness, spirit possession, oedema, prevention of disasters, sexually transmitted diseases and asthma. The study showed that the most common reasons for consulting a spiritualist are to help keep someone's love and to drive away evil spirits.

When medicine is given to a patient to "cure" any of the above illnesses or social problems, a ritual ceremony is usually performed at the healer's clinic to enhance the potency of the preparation. The patient is given advice on how to live with other members of the household, on how to take the medicine and on the correct food to eat. The patient is also asked to report back to the healer within a specified time, usually five days.

When asked how they were able to trace their patients or how they knew what had happened to them, the spiritualists replied that they knew their patients and had warned them to report if they encountered further problems. A few spiritualists kept records on their patients but the information they recorded was of a scanty nature, usually only names and addresses. They did not normally record the type of diagnosis or the type of treatment given.

Herbalists

Herbalists are the most numerous of the traditional healers. Their approach to healing is based on the use and application of herbs. Their methods of treatment and healing are often similar to those of modern medicine. Nevertheless, their techniques of healing cannot easily be explained by rational scientific enquiry. Herbalists use many techniques and procedures that are difficult to explain. There are various subspecialties within herbal medicine. Some herbalists specialize in bone treatment, others deal with cuts and others handle general medicine. Some sell herbal preparations, including love potions and medicine that protects against evil forces.

Of the herbalists interviewed during the period of fieldwork, many had their clinics in market-places, except in Eastern Province where herbalists and other traditional healers are not allowed to practise in the market. Those who practise their medicine in the open market often display herbs and other medicinal preparations for sale on large tables or on floor mats.

A herbalist sees the patient at the clinic which is often an open space by the market stall. At this clinic there may be chairs and a table. During the fieldwork it was noted that few patients called in the mornings to seek consultation. The peak consultation period was in the late afternoon when people were returning from work.

A herbalist deals with fewer patients than a modern health practitioner with an outpatient clinic. A herbalist sees about 20 patients a day and therefore has the advantage of having more time to talk with the patients. In a relaxed atmosphere a herbalist listens attentively to an account of the patient's problems, and asks questions about the patient's ailments, mental state and relationship with relatives.

When preliminary investigations have been conducted, the herbalist will examine the patient before prescribing treatment, touching the patient to find out if there are abnormalities on the body and enquiring if there is any pain. When the herbalist is satisfied that the patient's complaints can be dealt with, he or she reassures the patient not to worry. After payment of a consultation fee equivalent to about US$ 1, the herbalist prescribes treatment. Patients may also buy medicine without seeking advice.

A herbalist may perform the roles of counsellor, advising the patient, and of pharmacist. In addition, he or she is seen as a social worker who talks with patients and their relatives about life's problems.

The problems commonly dealt with by herbalists are love problems, marital discord, epilepsy, coughs, rheumatism, persistent headaches, prolonged menstruation, abdominal pains, infertility, back pain, diarrhoea, gonorrhoea, vomiting, asthma, lumps, impotence, child delinquency, worms and spirit possession. Herbalists also provide charms for good luck.

Social characteristics of traditional healers

A sample was taken of traditional healers in Lusaka, representing each of the four main types of healers, in order to find out some of their social characteristics. Apart from the fact that all the TBAs were female, it was noted that 56% of the remaining traditional healers were male.

Most healers had about six years of formal education. Of those above the age of 50, especially in rural areas, many were illiterate.

The age analysis showed that 70% of the traditional healers were in the age group 45–64 years. None was below the age of 35. Age is respected in African societies; elderly persons are accorded respect because of the experience they have acquired. In modern medical practice, young persons often occupy positions of responsibility, but in traditional healing the healers are mature adults.

The place of traditional medicine in Zambia

Traditional medicine appears to perform important social and medical functions, particularly with regard to psychosomatic problems. The healers treat people who are dissatisfied with modern medical treatment or who live in places where there are no modern medical institutions as the first line of contact. The common types of illness dealt with are in the domain of mental illness, alcohol dependence, poisoning, provision of "good luck", personality disorders, infertility, impotence and un-explained symptoms. These activities predate the primary health care programme and have been accorded official recognition thanks to steps taken by the Ministry of Health.

Whatever one may think of the effectiveness of traditional medicine, it continues to be important. In many situations the traditional healer is the first contact with the person seeking medical care. Traditional medi-cine is rooted in the community, the healer lives with the people in the community and the traditional health care is available in the community. In contrast, modern medicine has its origins and philosophy outside the community, the physician or nurse may be perceived as having little in common with the people of the community, and the health care is often available only after a lengthy and inconvenient journey. While the physician is a stranger in an unfamiliar clinic in a distant town, the herbalist may have a clinic at a stall in the local market-place.

It should be appreciated that to initiate and maintain primary health care in the community one has to build on traditional founda-tions. This factor, rather than legislation, seems to be the key to success-ful implementation of primary health care.

One of the concerns of the 1977 workshop on traditional medicine in primary health care was the possibility of regulating fees charged by traditional healers. It was suggested that if traditional healers could play their role within the national health care system a proportion of their fees could be redirected to the financing of national health care. It was estimated at that time that Zambians were spending up to US$ 28 million a year on traditional medicine, which was equivalent to 40% of the government's budget for health care. However tempting the prospect, the reality has proved illusory. There is a basic difference between the two systems of health care which makes it impossible to integrate traditional medicine and traditional healers (with the exception, perhaps, of TBAs) into a health care system based on modern medicine.

The Zambian experience has been that it is not possible to apply the scientific criteria of modern medicine to traditional medicine or traditional healers. The person who seeks the help of traditional medicine (again with the exception of the woman giving birth) is in many cases trying to find out which person or what spirit caused the illness, or which supernatural powers can put it right, or perhaps the patient is simply seeking reassurance and direction from a respected counsellor. The concerns are in most cases fundamentally different from those of the person who consults a medical practitioner in a modern health care system.

While the Zambian Government's system of primary health care is based on the principles of modern medicine, traditional medicine is founded on faith. But while the idea of being healed through having faith that one will be healed is intriguing, faith by very definition does not lend itself to medical scrutiny, which demands scientific evidence as proof. The lack of scientific medical standards precludes traditional healing from becoming part of Zambia's primary health care system based on the principles of modern medicine; but this does not mean that traditional healers should be ignored. On the contrary, experience in Zambia shows that they can be recognized for the important role they play in individual and community health. Accepted by the community and believed to provide a certain measure of success, traditional healers offer what might be described as their own primary health care system in Zambia — and particularly in rural Zambia — parallel to that provided by the medical authorities. There can be recognition of the parallel system of primary health care. There can be respect for the parallel system for it can indeed be successful. There can be assistance to the parallel system to help traditional healers heal more effectively. But integration of the belief system of traditional medicine with the scientific rigour of modern medicine was found in most cases to be impossible in Zambia, the exception being when herbs are tested scientifically and found to be effective.

There is plenty of scope for fruitful cooperation based on mutual respect. Zambia sees the need for dialogue with traditional healers in order to improve their services and avoid harmful practices. Traditional healers may be supported so that they may make their contribution to the health of the nation in their own way and so that their activities can be regulated. They can be provided with training and retraining courses, and those who satisfactorily complete such courses may perhaps be able to play a role in some formal primary health care programmes. TBAs must also be trained so that they can improve their midwifery knowledge and skills. This may be a positive way to improve health care delivery programmes, especially in rural areas.

CHAPTER 10

Looking back: lessons learned

J.M. Kasonde & J. D. Martin

The foregoing chapters have examined selected aspects of primary health care policy and practice in Zambia over more than a decade. The activities are those of government agents, NGOs and the community. They relate to problems of management as much as to those of resource availability. But they also point to lessons that are to be learned from the early years of primary health care and to suggestions for future strategies.

Community participation

Not surprisingly the greatest number of issues appear to have arisen around the communities themselves.

Community participation in planning appears to have been at best inadequate. Lowther and Moonde (Chapter 3) in their description of the Luangwa project go as far as stating that the project was imposed on the community. Oxfam's experience (Chapter 4) confirms this view. Community participation is crucial to the success of primary health care programmes. It is therefore important to attempt to find out why this element was lacking in spite of attempts to involve the community. To do this one must consider the perspectives of those concerned—the government, the community and the NGOs.

The Government of Zambia, through the Ministry of Health, clearly saw its duty as the provision of health care. Health workers would educate the community on the importance of clean water. Health workers would get the people to sink so many wells and dig so many latrines. The perception of the Ministry of Health as the provider seems to be the first obstacle to true community participation.

The community also perceived the Ministry of Health as provider and itself as recipient. This provider–recipient relationship derives from the doctor–patient relationship and is reinforced by the emphasis on medical care as opposed to health care and by the fact that physicians are the leaders of the health team. This perception by the community of itself as recipient is deeply ingrained in society and is incompatible with true community participation.

NGOs, on the other hand, appear to be the victims of a different phenomenon—the "project mentality". To the Ministry of Health they represent a source of funds for carrying out one project in the Ministry's programme of many activities. To the community they are a benevolent donor concerned with solving just one problem of many. The project will come and go, or more ominously it will be brought and taken away. That is why it belongs neither to the Ministry of Health nor to the community and that is why it is also incompatible with true community participation.

It appears from the experiences described that the three willing partners in this venture, in addition to taking the great care already shown in involving the community, need to do something more to foster community participation. First, there is a need to reorient the line of accountability. As long as the health worker has to account to the Ministry of Health rather than to the local council he or she will not be able adequately to foster community participation. At the same time existing local structures such as councils should reorient their perceptions both of themselves and of external agents. The issue lies in the way society is organized in general, not just in health care. Research into the nature and extent of these perceptions would be useful to health planners.

Apart from the problem of perceptions there is also the effect of limited resources. In theory it would seem that health care would be given priority in the allocation of resources where poverty prevails. In practice food and water supply are the first considerations of poor communities. Hunger is a more urgent problem than the prospect of illness. This tendency should be used to promote the health value of food and water supply. The primary health care worker may, in such situations, do more for health by joining in the production of food and provision of water than by urging the construction of a health facility. Similarly a community concerned about housing problems may be better served by help in building suitable shelter. Collaboration in health matters at community level should be determined by local priorities rather than by preoccupation with medical problems.

The health system

An important aspect of the observations on management of primary health care is the relationship between the organizational structure of the health system and that of primary health care. Several issues arise.

The impression is given that primary health care was one of many vertical programmes of the Ministry of Health. Thus one talks of the Primary Health Care Secretariat at the Ministry of Health, the primary health care teams in the district and the community health worker in the village. In other cases reference is made to the primary health care project at a given place. The effect of this is to compartmentalize a programme which ought to permeate the whole health care system. There is a strong case for re-examining the whole structure and the place of primary health care within it. Indeed, there is a need to share a common definition of primary health care since the concept seems to have been interpreted differently by different groups.

The primary health care strategy relies on a team structure; the assumption that the existing team structure could serve the new strategy should be re-examined.

Yet another concern is how to integrate an urgent vertical programme into the system without distorting the horizontal primary health care base. This happened in many cases with the advent of AIDS. A new and urgent challenge was thrust upon the health service and external funding was attracted to this emergency. The experience of Chikankata as described by Malama (Chapter 6) demonstrates that it is not only possible to incorporate a vertical programme in primary health care but that it can even be used to strengthen primary health care.

Decentralization of responsibility to district and community levels appears to be essential for successful implementation of primary health care. However, the difficulty of devolving responsibility without devolving financial control limited the extent to which decisions could be made locally. It was not within the power of the Ministry of Health alone to devolve financial control and other administrative responsibilities. The health system had to operate within the overall national administrative structure. It would also be good to see more community-initiated projects which do not rely on government instruction even if technical support comes from governmental agencies.

Intersectoral collaboration appears to have been given a low profile in the primary health care activities described. There are two reasons for this. First, reporting of activities by health workers tends to emphasize those factors directly relevant to the health sector such as the number of immunizations or clinic visits. Secondly, the outcomes normally used as indicators of progress in primary health care are direct health indicators such as morbidity and mortality. Improvements in food security or literacy are rarely demanded in the reports of health workers. There is a need to devise ways of reporting which assess health-related activities in a given area.

The observation by Macdonald (Chapter 5) that evaluation was not incorporated in the original design actually applies to many programmes. The enthusiasm for primary health care often leaves little room for a monitoring and evaluation plan. Yet this is of crucial importance if the cycle of planning, implementation and replanning is to be meaningful. Freund and Kalumba's description of a monitoring and evaluation study (Chapter 8) is therefore welcome. Their particular study looked at the process of community participation but evaluation of the inputs and outcomes could also be planned. For comparison it would be helpful if the procedures used in all primary health care evaluation activities were standardized. Studies on this subject should be correlated and an evaluation plan developed.

Evaluation, of course, should not be a "once-in-a-while" exercise but a continuous process in which activities are constantly and systematically scrutinized with a focus on the objectives meant to be attained.

Financing primary health care

All the authors agree that one of the obstacles to the implementation of primary health care is the lack of resources. This shortage is seen formally in the failure to obtain building materials, drugs and other essentials as well as informally in the failure of communities to support community health workers. It is therefore necessary to address issues of financing for primary health care.

The period under review was a time of economic stagnation or decline in Zambia. There was therefore a corresponding decline in resources available to the health sector overall. Further, within the health sector, the marginalization of primary health care activities had the effect of limiting the budgetary allocation to primary health care. Moreover, in an environment which emphasized "free health services" as a principle, it was difficult to sustain a programme based on payment for services at community level.

It appears that four developments would be required for the financing of primary health care to increase: an improvement in the national economy, an increase in the health sector share of that economy, an increase in the primary health care share of health sector resources, and a more favourable attitude to income generation or cost recovery. Since the improvement in national economic output is outside the sphere of influence of the health worker, only the other three issues are discussed here.

There is a strong case for increasing the health sector's share of the national budget. This increase need only be small in medical services but it should be much greater in health promotion activities. It is suggested that the stimulation of health promotion activities in the agriculture, education and community development sectors requires more formal support. Similarly, within the health system primary health care strategies and activities should permeate health programmes. This incorporation of primary health care in the totality of the health system is the essential element in increasing financial support.

The generation of resources for primary health care is a more complex issue. Current experience shows that it is possible to generate funds and other resources locally but that these sources are uneven and cannot be relied on to sustain a long-term programme. The provision of health care free to all was a measure of equity, but its effect has been to create inertia whenever a situation calling for payment has arisen. If payment is going to be accepted as a strategy for financing primary health care it will have to be established as such in the whole health care system. The immediate need, however, is for a rational basis for income generation. There should be an analysis of requirements for capital and recurrent expenditure at community level, a long-term budget and an assessment of what the community can reasonably be expected to raise as a contribution to both. There should also be clearly defined channels for accounting for revenue and expenditure.

The contribution of NGOs to this resource mobilization effort deserves special mention. NGOs have a very important role in the implementation of primary health care in developing countries. They have the advantage of being able to establish direct contact with communities. Because of their importance it is essential that they avoid certain factors that may make their efforts counterproductive.

The first of these factors is the "project mentality". The activities of NGOs may be viewed as time-limited external projects which are not part of the community's long-term health care plans. For this reason NGO activities may not get the commitment of the local community. It is essential that an understanding of local organizational structures precedes implementation so that the project becomes identified with local efforts. The message is that the project is being supported not because local people cannot do it but because they can do better with some help what they had already been doing and will continue to do. The second factor may be described as "competitive inhibition". The infusion of external resources and ideas inhibits local initiative. An instance of this is the reduction of government input when NGO resources became available as reported in the Eastern Province. This inhibition of local initiative can be prevented if participation in the planning process is active rather than passive. The third risk is that of distorting priorities. Large external inputs to a particular primary health care project may distract attention from other aspects. An example would be a large project on sanitation and its effect on, for instance, child immunization in a given area.

These and other constraints are not insurmountable, however, and should not detract from the fact that NGOs, both foreign and local, have a major role in the implementation of national primary health care programmes. NGOs have shown their capacity to fill gaps. They must be encouraged.

Traditional medicine

The studies of Professor Twumasi (Chapter 9) confirm that a majority of Zambian society has a deep-seated belief in traditional medicine. As he points out, traditional medicine operates as a parallel health system. The question of integration therefore does not arise if this means absorption into the "modern" medical system. Integration is necessary and appropriate when this refers to recognition and support within the totality of the health sector, the latter term referring to all health and health-care-related activities in the country. Viewed in this light, traditional medicine becomes one of a group of systems that have as a common objective the promotion of the health of the community and of individuals.

Twumasi has dealt with the validity of traditional healing in terms of widespread community acceptance and the practical relief that it can offer to individuals. The obvious next step is to devise the rules and regulations under which the system can operate without causing harm. This involves much more than the determination of fees and the listing of recognized healers. It requires in-depth study of criteria for evaluating services and the balance of risk and benefit. It also requires research into the foundations of practices, whether in terms of modern biomedical understanding or in terms of cultural and psychological support.

Primary health care and the individual

The deliverer–recipient attitude that pervades primary health care activities tends to lay inadequate emphasis on the role of the individual in personal or family health care. A strong case seems to have emerged for targeting the individual and defining the role he or she is expected to play.

A useful exercise might have been a study of the perception of individuals regarding the concept of primary health care and how it related to the established health care system. This would have at least three advantages. Firstly, since the policy-makers are part of the community it would ensure a favourable attitude among them. Secondly, it would provide a receptive audience for the approaches of health workers who deliver the programme. Finally, it would create motivation for individuals to play their part in primary health care as contributors to communal and personal health promotion activities. Ultimately the individual is both the main target and the main promoter of primary health care.

Development of human resources for primary health care

The basic assumption underlying all the experiences described is that there are adequate human resources, of the appropriate type, to deliver the primary health care programme. Yet it is clear that the human resources element was the most difficult to satisfy. Inadequate attention seems to have been paid to the reorientation of health workers to the new strategy. This omission may have had a more obstructing effect than was apparent.

The creation of community health workers was a key development in the whole programme. Yet problems have been highlighted regarding their capacity to operate. Community support, financial and otherwise, was often not forthcoming or was irregular. Experience points to the need for a clearer definition of the role and functions of community health workers who are an essential link between the community and the formal health system.

Teamwork, or the lack of it, has been highlighted. The need has been identified for reorientation of health workers and their role in the teams that manage primary health care.

Detailed plans were laid for the progressive training of physicians, nurses and other health workers but the planned output was not achieved and the necessary redistribution of nursing personnel was not carried out. The effect of these constraints, and that of an unexpected exodus of physicians, was to weaken the referral and supervisory systems and therefore primary health care itself. However, lack of reorientation of some health workers was an even greater constraint. The reorientation and fuller involvement of senior health workers are urgently needed.

Technical assistance

Many agencies, governmental and nongovernmental, recognized the need to contribute to primary health care. Much national support to the programme was in fact a conveyance of external funds. The place of technical assistance still needs to be evaluated.

The availability of a strategic plan, setting out in one document the intentions of the Ministry of Health in promoting primary health care, made it possible for donors to identify aspects of particular interest to them. However, the sporadic nature of this support made it difficult to budget well in advance. A number of criteria seem to be essential for optimal external support to primary health care. These include the timely indication of intention to support the programme, long-term commitment and some degree of flexibility in adjusting to changing circumstances. Another useful area not often recognized as worthy of support is research and evaluation. Technical assistance to primary health care needs to be increased within the context of nationally determined strategies.

Research needs

A clear need has emerged for research on many aspects of the implementation of primary health care as a prerequisite for sound planning of future activities. Urgent research areas would appear to be both operational and fundamental.

Questions to be answered through operational research include problems of teamwork, supervision and logistic support. The health care chain should now be dissected to identify constraints at all links and to suggest solutions on a continuing basis. The causes of such constraints as lack of support for community health workers, low motivation for community service and lack of interest by some health workers should be identified.

Fundamental issues for study would include perceptions of primary health care by health workers and communities, current systems and structures of social ·organization, the impact of health education, and epidemiological patterns of ill-health. In both the operational and fundamental investigations, as much attention should be paid to successful outcomes as to unsuccessful ones and a link to the decision-making process should be established so that results are fed into the process as soon as they are available.

The way forward

The issues raised in the preceding chapters apply not only to Zambia but also to other developing countries. If there is a single lesson to be learned from these experiences it is that the introduction of a major strategy such as primary health care requires more than the addition of a project to an existing health system. It involves a complete reorientation of the organizational and management structure of the system.

The strategies of the future must take account of the place of primary health care within the health system, community participation and resource mobilization. The place of primary health care as a horizontal strategy permeating all health programmes has yet to be established fully. Development of mechanisms to achieve this pose a challenge to the leadership of the future. Active community participation, though recognized as essential by all concerned, requires further strengthening to ensure that primary health care becomes a normal part of social organization at all levels. The mechanisms required to achieve this constitute a second challenge to the leadership. As for resource mobilization, it appears that all three aspects of income generation, technical assistance and rational utilization need more attention. The department responsible for resource mobilization should be much increased, commensurate with the task ahead.

Following the elections in Zambia in 1991, the new government set about a reorientation of the health care system that addresses many of the concerns dealt with here. Progress so far indicates that a number of necessary measures have been implemented and others are under way. Decentralization of responsibility and accountability, together with cost recovery, are basic to the newly emerging system. In the final chapter of this book, a team from the Zambian Ministry of Health describes its vision for future health care and frankly confronts a number of controversial issues. It is their vision that will be the foundation for Zambia's health care system, rooted in a primary health care approach, for the next century.

CHAPTER 11

Looking forward: Zambia's health system reform agenda into the next century

K. Kalumba, E. Nangawe, L. M. Muuka-Kalumba & V. Musowe

The search for concepts

Achievement depends on a shared vision of a preferred future that is not simply stumbled into but deliberately chosen. This must be a morally preferred vision, chosen not just because it seeks to make things better for us today but rather because it forces us to take tough decisions now to carry out our collective responsibility to ensure the positive interests of future generations.

Strategic health planning based upon a strategic health vision serves a known social purpose. A scenario for a healthy future for Zambia cannot be derived from a trend planning exercise on how many hospitals the country is going to have, how much will be spent on drugs or, indeed, how many doctors are going to be trained or attracted back from abroad. Nor indeed is it enough to simply say we need health for all. The questions of what is the preferred health state of Zambians and what issues must be resolved to achieve that state are crucial to a future definition of health in Zambian society.

Because we live in an age of rapid change, our vision of the future must include a sense of social consciousness. We face issues such as how to deal with poverty, poor housing conditions, sanitation and nutrition. We must cope with population growth, new or resurgent problems such as AIDS and malaria, and rapid political transformation towards democracy. All these factors make planning for health reform in any sub-Saharan African country difficult.

The core concepts underlying Zambia's health sector reform were described in the policy framework paper for the Movement for Multi-Party Democracy (MMD) Presidential Advisory Group. The paper was prepared well before the October 1991 democratic elections, which led to a major political transformation of the country from a one-party state to a pluralist democracy in Zambia's Third Republic. Underlying the thinking of the framework paper were lessons learned from many years of study of health reforms in Zambia and other countries. A key concern was that the limits of past reforms were not primarily medical/technical but rather political and managerial.

The dynamics of the status quo

Past practices have left Zambia with a health care system characterized by:

— erosion of the infrastructure
— declining access to health services
— increased malnutrition
— inadequate supply of drugs
— increased infant mortality
— poor staff morale, with many professionals leaving the country.

Even more fundamental than these symptoms are the constraints that frustrated many efforts at reform in the past and could continue to do so in the future if a new approach is not followed. Characteristically, health planners, lacking a social vision for health, have resorted to the practice of strategic planning. But this practice, typical of many health development plans of the past, becomes planning for its own sake. Witness the observation of Dr JFC Haslam, Director of Medical Services from 1933 to 1946, as he introduced his Ten-Year Health Services Development Plan (1945–1955):

> Sitting down, at the age of fifty-seven, to write the memorandum on development of health services in Northern Rhodesia ... it seems certain that I shall never carry out the plans, dearly as I should like to do so. Like others who have done a great deal of planning, I have been at times somewhat cast down when many hours of work and thought have served no more useful purpose than to swell the bulk of a file called Health Department Future Development. Like others too, I have smiled sadly when turning the yellowing pages of an ancient file recording the plans of a predecessor which, after a full, careful and hopeful period of gestation, either failed at delivery and died *in utero* or succumbed soon after birth to the east wind of financial stringency.

Haslam's plan suffered the same fate that many attempts at reform in the health sector suffered many years after colonial rule.

In order for Zambia to become one of the healthiest nations a new health vision is necessary. This vision has to be evolved in a situation that is influenced by several pre-existing issues, such as:

— lack of societal consensus on future directions in health care;
— social and health care systems that focus on care of the sick rather than emphasize health;
— the extent to which the health system is driven by medical professional demands for new and expensive technology;
— increased pressures resulting from a rapidly changing social, demographic, political, macroeconomic and physical environment;
— the extent to which short-term economic considerations dominate decision-making;
— the way in which jurisdictional and ministerial boundaries inhibit actions that would foster good health.

97

Zambia's health care system has developed over the years essentially as a sickness care system. The services provided, including education, research, planning and data collection, are all focused on illness and disease. This orientation on sickness is coupled with ignorance of alternative practices and other approaches. The Zambian medical education system appears to produce "medical technologists" but few health scientists and health care professionals trained to look beyond "disease" to a wider concept of health. The colonial basis of this deficiency is well documented.

Overall levels of financial support for health promotion and illness prevention have characteristically been too low for the development of appropriate services or innovations. Relegated to local government municipalities as part of a colonial heritage, the community (public) health interventions relevant to disease prevention have been hampered from taking major initiatives by limited resources, inadequate legislative powers and weak management leadership.

There has always been a lack of coordination between health, finance (especially macroeconomic planning) and social services at the policy and programme levels. Furthermore, government decisions in various ministries are not assessed with respect to their impact on community health.

In all past reform efforts, it was clear that there was difficulty in securing broader ownership of the reform idea of strategic planning for new health policies within the Ministry of Health (see Chapter 2). Past neglect in building consumer responsibility for health, lack of conceptual clarity and initiative among medical professionals in management leadership, and the absence of other relevant disciplines at top management and other professional levels—including health economists, health policy analysts and others—have led to deficiencies in key decision-making.

The weak legislative position of the Ministry of Health has always weakened public legitimation of reform plans. Until now, the most comprehensive health reform legislation was the 1930 Public Health Ordinance. No comprehensive review of legislation has been done since then to make regulations consistent with a clear vision of a healthy future. At no time during major reform attempts, such as the Haslam Plan of 1945–55, the 1972 Ten-Year Health Plan, or indeed the primary health care initiatives of the 1980s, was initiative taken to carry out major legislative reform in line with the changes proposed. There is ample evidence that existing legislation was often at odds with reform. Initiatives such as the Medical Services Act of 1985 were not only piecemeal but contradicted the Public Health Act. The Medical Services Act was really a hospital boards act. In the absence of effective legislation on reform, public decision-making and programmes were developed on the basis of institutional aspirations or professional demands rather than the needs of the community.

There was a need to address the political implications of cost containment and cost recovery which were inevitable if quality health care was to be assured. Further, the institutional prerequisites for cost recovery, such as unit costs of services and collection and retention mechanisms, needed to be worked out.

The scarcity of resources increased pressures for new revenue sources to complement state budgets. Proposals for a Social Security and National Health Insurance scheme became stuck in bureaucratic inertia that indicated lack of technical skills to appraise its merits and demerits. Further, the fee-for-service system that was sporadically implemented, particularly in church-run rural medical institutions, was seen to be biased towards the provision of "cures" rather than health promotion and illness prevention. This inevitably encouraged the greater use of institutional services. In addition, fears about equity were being raised in relation to proposals for recovering costs. Zambian political and medical leaders had to be fully educated on the need for a new paradigm on health development.

It is clear that increased demands for new and expensive technologies in Zambia's health care were made with little or no assessment of efficacy. Poor policies and procedures for maintenance of equipment in hospitals and health centres coupled with unskilled use have led to a waste of useful technology. Moreover, dependence on technological solutions reinforced the bias towards the medical model and promoted the overspecialization of professionals. These, lacking sophisticated equipment in Zambian hospitals, drifted away to "greener pastures" as soon as they completed training abroad. The high costs associated with technological solutions resulted in a shift of resources away from community-focused caring programmes. There was a need to define a basic package of essential health services.

Bureaucratic inertia made it difficult to achieve change that was both politically inspired and scientifically correct. Consequently, new initiatives received little encouragement from Ministry of Health officials.

Because of the recession and fiscal policy rationalization, various community support services had already begun to suffer. Inefficient administration of the social welfare fund created credibility problems for the MMD government's plan to create social safety nets while carrying out economic restructuring. The result was that economic reforms had to be distorted in order to be acceptable. Hence their outcome, as well as their impact on health, became in the process unpredictable.

Defining a vision of health into the 21st century

Underlying Zambia's current health reform effort is a very specific definition of health. We understand health to mean the extent to which an individual or group is able, on the one hand, to realize aspirations and satisfy needs and, on the other hand, to change or cope with the environment. Health is therefore seen as a resource for everyday life, not the objective of living; it is a positive concept emphasizing social and personal resources as well as physical capacity. Health is therefore threatened when people's overall quality of life declines or, to express it in another way, when their misery index is high.

From this concept of health are derived three core aims for health intervention. These represent our vision of health in the future. Thus health sector strategies must lead to a society in which Zambians:

— create environments conducive to health
— learn the art of being well
— provide basic health care for all.

Zambia's commitment to provision of better management for quality health care for the individual, the family and the community, was under-lined in the 1992 document *National health policies and strategies (health reforms)*. This document is based on the following policy package:

— a goal-oriented, financially sound management system for health care;
— clear accountability and responsibilities at every level;
— a mechanism for regular review of progress;
— enhancement of the role and responsibilities of consumers;
— strengthening of community-based health care supported by health centres;
— maintenance of the role of public hospitals, including pyschiatric hospitals and the University Teaching Hospital;
— integration of private sector strengths and resources;
— improvement of quality assurance and treatment effectiveness;
— a broader range of professionally regulated health providers (includ-ing biomedical technicians, nurses, mental health professionals and other social health and cultural-medical healers), with improved conditions of service and stronger teamwork in both clinical and public health settings.

This policy package was translated into health goals which underpin the whole document. Zambia's goals are:

Goal 1   To achieve equity in health opportunities
Goal 2   To increase the life expectancy of Zambians
Goal 3   To create environments that support health
Goal 4   To encourage lifestyles that support health
Goal 5   To provide quality health services
Goal 6   To promote public policies that support health
Goal 7   To improve individual and family health through efficiently administered population control activities.

These goals are fully elaborated in terms of specific interventions.

This vision for health translates into the Ministry of Health's Mission Statement in which the Zambian Government has stated its commitment to developing a health care system that will provide Zambians with equity of access to cost-effective quality health care as close to the family as possible.

It is important to state that there is sometimes confusion, even among the Ministry's technical officials, between our vision of health for society and the Ministry of Health's Mission Statement aimed at making that vision reality.

One concept in the Ministry of Health's Mission Statement requires elaboration. Equity of health policies has always been a difficult concept. Our understanding is that equity means that no group or individual receives less than a minimum benefit level or more than a maximum cost level of health care. We can thus talk in terms of equity of health benefits or equity of health costs. Hence, in terms of access to health care, a basic health package for all that is optimally costed for users minimizes constraints on equity while allowing for those who can afford higher-cost services to have that choice on the principle of individual responsibility for health.

Equity of access to cost-effective quality health care depends on a combination of efficiency, effectiveness and equity. Society has several choices. A society may, for instance, allocate benefits more equitably by increasing the amount of benefits, or by reducing the population, or by diluting the level of benefits. And a society may distribute costs more evenly by decreasing the total cost burden, by widening the population base of those who contribute in order to spread the costs, or by raising the cost level that members of society are willing to accept.

Major structural reform

The major thrust of health reforms has been in devolution of the key Ministry of Health functions of planning, management, service delivery, funding/resource allocation and revenue generation. These have been complemented by strategic reforms to foster strong commitment from central government and others already involved, clear goals and objectives, clear definition of roles and responsibilities backed by a legislative reform agenda and corporate planning. In addition, issues such as gender and health, human resource development, the role of NGOs and donor co-ordination have been addressed.

Establishing autonomous health boards

Decentralization—so that districts and major hospital authorities can have discretionary authority for personnel recruitment, the assignment of tasks and allocation of resources—has been a central focus of health system reform. This process includes the need to set up suitable structures for community participation in decision-making, for quality control and for financial accountability. As decentralization gets under way, the central administration is pressed to increase its capacity for monitoring and consultation.

The role of the Ministry of Health headquarters is being transformed into a Central Board of Health with the objective of building up its capacity to provide the following:

— a pool of expertise in the major departments of health planning and management, personnel, clinical services, basic health programmes, logistics and technical support and administration;
— capacity building for management initiatives in district-based health care;
— a structure that will ensure the ability to monitor the quality of health care;
— improved financing for the health sector.

This new central structure makes the relationship between central policy-makers, ministers and the professional–technical operations of the central board clearer. Other responsibilities of the central administration are being rationalized. These include the setting of policies and national guidelines, coordination of research and provision of information on health issues, and coordination of donor contributions to the health sector.

While the initial policy priorities have been formulated by the centre, it is the eventual aim of the reform process that the districts will provide plans conceived by their district management teams and approved by the district health boards for incorporation into an annual national plan. New projects and programmes which fall within the context of the reform process are designed so that they can be realistically assessed. To ensure the feasibility of projects and programmes, information is gathered by the planners through pilot studies, and empirical data are collected and analysed by the health reform implementation teams. To ensure that this process is feasible at district level, the health reform implementation teams have embarked on a programme of management training in all the districts, and a private accountancy firm has also begun training at least one staff member from each district in new accounting and monitoring procedures. All this will help the district health management teams currently in place to play a more effective role in meeting the needs of their districts by identifying and prioritizing problems, formulating strategies for intervention, costing those interventions and evaluating their outcomes. What is evolving is a new structure of relationships between the central ministry and the districts.

Simultaneously with Ministry of Health reforms, autonomously managed District Health Boards are being established. These will be accountable in technical matters to the Ministry of Health but will be administratively part of the local government. While much of the work in the first part of 1993 focused on strengthening the district health management teams, the introduction of District Health Boards will strengthen the current process of decentralization. In this regard, all provinces have been visited to discuss and plan the formation of district and regional hospital boards. District Health Boards, through their technical teams, will carry out rapid assessments of their districts using epidemiological evidence to identify and prioritize problems. The District Health Boards will then formulate strategies for interventions and will cost the interventions before submitting budget proposals, after approval by district policy bodies, to the Ministry of Health. An evaluation and monitoring component will be included to help the districts see the effectiveness of their interventions.

As a measure of commitment to the district strategy, the health sector budget for 1994 is based on a weighted allocation of US$ 2 per capita. Priority has been given to district funding (8 billion Zambian kwacha, which is nearly 20% of the sector estimates) in this budget. If carried through, the 1994 budget will represent 13% of the total government budget, which clearly reflects a serious intention to invest in district health services.

The most crucial dimension of decentralization is the extent to which communities and families will benefit, as indicated in the Ministry's own Mission Statement. The District Health Boards will be able to carry out basic health programmes, such as those concerned with maternal and child health or malaria, and will also deal with localized problems such as dysentery or scabies outbreaks. The District Health Boards will be expected to set up Area Health Boards to be the link with health service users and to encourage quality control and community involvement.

Since district and health centre plans may be insufficient as they may not reflect people's inputs in the health planning process, a "Health Neighbourhood Watch" initiative has been proposed to encourage people's involvement.

A consultative group on building partnerships for the health reforms came into being at a special workshop on concepts and strategies. The workshop has helped throw some light on basic assumptions and risks inherent in the "Health Neighbourhood Watch" proposal.

Central Hospital Management Boards have been set up in all major hospitals and have the same legal status and relationship to the Ministry of Health as the District Health Boards.

The former Provincial Medical Officers have now become regional health advisers to the District Health Boards on matters such as annual plans and use of resources. The advisers will monitor progress and audit the accounts of the districts. They will also facilitate training to improve the provision of health care and ensure that the quality of health care is maintained. General hospitals at provincial level will have the same autonomy as the District Health Boards but will be directly accountable to the Ministry of Health.

Reforms in the financing of health

Zambia's health policies call for initiatives in the area of cost containment and sourcing of revenue. For example, effective cost containment requires a budget structure that would permit difficult options to be decided upon and would make possible the most effective provision of health services to a specific population. This has given rise to a radical health budget reform that required change in the budget practices of the Ministry of Finance. Through experimental pilot projects, the Ministry of Health budget reform team was able to show that cost containment and effective service provision were possible even at district level. Hence, starting from 1994, district health budgeting became a reality.

Financing the curative aspects of Zambia's health system has always been problematic. The long tradition of central budgets financed from public taxation yet with a narrow tax base in the country overall has, since the 1930s, frustrated equity-based strategic planning in the health sector. Our principle of building partnership for health has led us to reformulate the concept of equity. All able-bodied Zambians able to earn an income are, in principle, expected to contribute to the cost of health care at the same time as all persons are entitled to a minimum package of essential services. It is recognized that such a scheme does not provide total equity.

Since the formal publication of *National health policies and strategies (health reforms)* in 1992, there have been intensive discussions on options for raising more resources for the health sector. The main options highlighted in the reforms include:

— compulsory/private health insurance
— user charges (cost recovery and cost sharing)
— community financing.

The primary reason for discussion of these options is that Zambia finds itself no longer able to raise the additional revenue required to finance health services through taxation.

There have been five main arguments for cost sharing in the Zambian context. Firstly, it is believed that cost sharing prevents unnecessary or frivolous use of government services and thus ensures that the services the government subsidizes are the most cost-effective ones and that medical services in general are used by those in real need. Secondly, it is considered a basic economic tenet that most patients should pay, if only marginally, towards the cost of what is provided. This is consistent with the overall thrust of market reform in society in general.

Thirdly, patients already pay considerable sums to mission medical facilities and to traditional healers. The former are able to go a long way towards being self-supporting, at least in terms of recurrent costs, and the latter are wholly self-supporting, even if sometimes less effective in curing patients. From these comparisons it is argued that similar charges could be made for government services.

Fourthly, charges will provide finance that will enable services to be improved for all users. On the other hand, it has been argued that charges are bound to be inequitable as no effective way could be found to exempt the poor. Finally, Zambia believes that cost sharing goes a long way towards sustaining programmes or projects funded by donors.

The heterogeneity of the Zambian community (socially, culturally and economically) and health institutions in the national health system is reflected in the number of bodies that are involved in the financing and delivery of services.

In practice, the determination of appropriate methods of financing the health sector is complicated because the mechanisms are numerous, their operation often complex, and their effects multiple.

By upholding the policy position that all people should contribute towards good quality health care as a preferred future state, solutions have to be found to the many vexing questions relating to financing health care.

The Ministry of Health in Zambia has been studying a number of options for financing health care.

Rural social insurance option

Social insurance is conventionally financed by imposing mandatory insurance contributions on employees as a percentage of their wages and by imposing on their employers a similar or somewhat higher payroll tax.

The introduction of social insurance in urban areas may not be viable at a time when Zambia is facing the worst economic recession in living memory and formal employment accounts for only 3.9% of the economy. Instead, the Ministry of Health is actively pursuing a pilot project in the area of Mwase-Mphangwe that is designed to provide social insurance for rural areas. The idea is based on careful studies of similar experiments in countries such as India.

Under this social insurance option for rural areas the idea being pursued is that each farming community family that contributes a bag of produce towards its health maintenance will be issued with a "family health card" which would entitle it to access to health services for 12 months, anywhere in the country. Referrals and bills from other districts would be settled by the district where the family has its permanent residence. The logistics of this plan need further work at the moment. A proposal to provide social safety nets for the very poor is being developed in conjunction with the Ministry of Community Development and Social Welfare. This would apply to both rural and urban areas though with different criteria of eligibility.

Funds realized in each district would be retained by the District Health Board for improvement of the quality of health care.

The Ministry of Health considers the family health card scheme to be a viable option for Zambia because the community is built on a tradition of mutual aid. It has always been a Zambian tradition to pay for the services rendered by the traditional healers, even though payment is usually in the form of gifts to the healer. Moreover, since the community in the rural area is fairly stable, paying in kind is a logical option. There are, of course, many issues that still have to be tested, and outcomes cannot be predicted with certainty. Questions of equity, efficiency, logistics, coverage and acceptability are being tested. For example, in the pilot project area of Mwase-Mphangwe, bags of maize contributed by households were yet to be collected for market by early November because of confusion caused by the introduction of a new crop marketing system in 1993.

A mix of strategies for urban areas

Zambia is a highly urbanized country. A separate set of strategies are therefore called for in dealing with the urban population.

The health financing scheme for urban areas will cover those employed in both formal and informal sectors. The schemes will be based on a mix of both public and private insurance schemes. Direct user charges and earmarked taxes (both direct and indirect) will cover those who may opt out of insurance schemes.

The price (or "premium") charged for private health insurance will be based not on pooled risks but on personal risk characteristics. Premiums would vary for different individuals or groups. The scheme could be either for profit or non-profit, and would be organized for individuals or groups. Along the same line is a growing interest in the concept of health maintenance organizations. In connection with the private insurance scheme, the Ministry of Health would encourage the development of health maintenance organizations into which individuals or groups would contract. Established health maintenance organizations would cover all the health needs of members (either in the organization's own facilities or those under contract to it) in return for an annual payment. The integration of the insurance and provider functions would provide an incentive for cost containment in contrast to a third-party payment system.

In addition to the above scheme, employers will continue to finance health care directly for their employees. This will include paying for private sector health services, employing medical personnel directly, or providing necessary facilities and equipment. Services provided by employer-financed schemes will include general medical services, personal preventive services, environmental and sanitation services and occupational health. Employers would offer these services as a fringe benefit to their workers and, once established, the benefit would be difficult to withdraw. Although examples of this approach exist in the mining industry, more consultative work is needed before it is applied more generally.

General tax revenue is to provide major financing for the health sector. The tax revenue target would be not less than 11% of national income. Financial resources would be allocated to districts on the basis of a resource allocation formula. For 1994, for example, the Ministry of Health has used a per capita allocation formula. Future ideas under consideration include a needs index.

The allocation of financial resources to districts for the implementation of a basic package of health care would continue to be one of the main functions of the Ministry of Health headquarters.

Household income is ultimately the source of most health care finance, but direct expenditures constitute a specific category of financing. Included in this category are any payments health consumers make directly (such as user charges) to health providers. Government health care services will charge user fees (which will be nominal) for specified services to health consumers not covered by social or private health insurance schemes. Even with insurance coverage, there would be a requirement for some degree of user payment.

Furthermore, traditional healers and purchase of pharmaceuticals are important examples of direct household expenditure on health.

The nationwide introduction of user fees in major health institutions followed many years of "free" medical provision. In introducing user fees the Ministry of Health worked out careful guidelines aimed at balancing its major principles and goals. The guidelines have been disseminated both to health workers and to the public. The Ministry of Health is continuously studying patterns of health service use.

Donor funds

The Ministry of Health and donors have noted that at all levels there is poor accountability for funds. Responsibility has been laid at the doors of both the Ministry of Health and the donors. Too often there have been poor policies, poor project and programme design, weak coordination and hidden agendas carried over from the past. The Ministry of Health has taken the lead in changing this process by focusing on capacity building, health policy reform and research.

Five main factors influence the extent to which programmes and projects supported by donor funds can be monitored effectively.

Firstly, there is the kind of agreement entered into with the donor partner. There are bilateral agreements that are held on a quarterly basis, as is the case with the Swedish International Development Authority and WHO; there are agreements that are held on an annual basis; and there are ad hoc agreements that are made as requests and offers come up. The type of agreement that is easiest to monitor in terms of funds is the bilateral agreement that specifies the amounts, the patterns of disbursal and the time period. The donor and the Ministry of Health are both bound by the terms of the agreement and can change or reallocate resources only by having further discussions and reaching consensus. The kind of aid that is most difficult to monitor is that which bypasses the Ministry of Finance and Ministry of Health headquarters and goes directly to programmes and projects. In this case the Ministry of Health has to rely on the programme manager to provide detailed accounts of income and expenditures to its accounts section. Often accounting procedures may be unsatisfactory because of lack of proper training, lack of guidelines, lack of logistic support and other problems.

Secondly, there is the manner in which the funds have been disbursed — whether through the Ministry of Finance, through the Bank of Zambia or directly to the projects and programmes. If aid is provided through the Bank of Zambia or the Ministry of Finance, there is the possibility to double-check total amounts disbursed. This may not always be the case with funds that go directly to the programmes since the Ministry of Finance will have no knowledge of them and they will not be reflected in national budget estimates, the Public Investment Programme or the Public Expenditure Review until the following year, and even then only if the Ministry of Health can obtain these data from the programmes. Health funds disbursed through the office of the Provincial Permanent Secretary may be reallocated for other activities or to other ministries, and there is no way that this can be controlled unless the funds are given either to the Provincial Medical Officer, as in the past, or directly to the districts.

Thirdly, the manner in which the planning process is organized also affects monitoring. If the monitoring component is not considered in the planning phase, it will not be seen as a priority and will be difficult to implement after the programme or project has already begun.

Fourthly, monitoring may be influenced by the various obligations of the donors to their own governments. Most donors have strict procedures they must follow regarding their own accountability for funds. If the supported programme or project does not have a monitoring component, then it is likely that the donor body will arrange its own monitoring. Donors may share their report findings with Zambia's Ministry of Health, but there have been instances where external consultants have been engaged to carry out monitoring and evaluation and the reports are not always written in English. The reports are usually provided to the programme managers and are not always shared widely or incorporated in Ministry of Health records. The indicators used for monitoring are not always the ones the Ministry of Health would have desired.

A fifth factor that may influence monitoring of programmes and projects is the capacity of Ministry of Health staff accurately to record information on expenditures at district, provincial and headquarters levels. If health personnel charged with financial monitoring lack the skills or the material and other resources to carry out their work, then one can expect poor results. There must be clear and concise guidelines as to how the information should be obtained and transmitted to Ministry of Health headquarters.

In the past, the Ministry of Health did not make systematic attempts to coordinate donor operations as a means of mobilizing assistance. While the government requested external assistance on occasion, a number of donors preferred to scout around for areas to support, using their own staff or consultants to carry out feasibility studies. Once satisfied with a proposal, they would ask the Government of Zambia for the go-ahead, which included asking the government to provide personnel and, sometimes, accommodation for expatriate staff. For those donors who chose to work specifically at district level, as did many voluntary agencies, it was often the case that Ministry of Health headquarters would not be aware of their activities since they were sanctioned directly by the National Commission for Development Planning, the designated agency for technical cooperation. While donors would carry out reporting and accounting according to their own needs, the information would not be made available to the Ministry of Health for incorporation in government health expenditures and thus resulted in under-reporting. Such projects and programmes created dependency, lack of sustainability and the ultimate collapse of health service provision once donor funding ceased.

Some donor coordination was provided in 1990–91 through the meetings of the health group of the Social Action Programme. In turn, the donors would hold occasional meetings convened by the "lead donor", the Netherlands. The term "lead donor" then was applied to a donor that coordinated the activities of other donors within the Social Action Programme. Now the term is applied to the coordination role within specific programmes and projects, such as when a donor commits itself to making a major contribution to a programme and takes the lead role of coordinating the work of other donors interested in the same area of support. Zambia's national health policy acknowledges the crucial importance of donor funding for the development of the health sector, and the need for coordination to involve donors in planning and progress reviews. The Ministry of Health now holds donor coordination meetings regularly to ensure donor support to the implementation of health reforms. An update on progress is given and donors are asked to consider those areas where assistance is still needed.

There has been an extremely positive response from donors supporting the health sector and there are even "new" donors entering the sector as a result of the reform of health policy. As a result of improved donor coordination, it is easier to keep track of donor pledges and commitments, and the relationship between the Ministry of Health and donors is generally warm. This coordination should be nurtured and encouraged to grow further. To enhance financial monitoring and follow-up, the Ministry of Health is considering a more effective and efficient information system created by the Division of Environmental Health of WHO. To help improve data collection in the districts, a new form of financial reporting is currently being tested. The overall aim is to make sure each district is able to provide accurate data on expenditures that can then be incorporated into the national health reports.

According to Zambia's national health policy, one of the Ministry of Health's responsibilities is to coordinate donor contributions. In this regard, the Ministry has complete autonomy in dealing directly with donors at both headquarters and programme level. However, for easy monitoring of assistance the Ministry would like to ensure that all assistance is first noted by the National Commission for Development Planning which is technically responsible for formal agreements. While the government has considerable control over the preparation of programme proposals, influence over donor consideration and acceptance depends on a number of issues.

Donors have their own priorities that influence to a certain extent their preferred areas of assistance. As many writers have indicated, the variables in allocating resources may be of a health, economic or political nature, or a combination of these. For example, indicators determining support could be based on infant and child mortality rates, or on the political system, or on per capita income, or on population levels. Many donors have specific programmes they wish to support and have allocated funds for these — such as HIV/AIDS programmes, the Essential Drugs Programme, immunization and, less frequently, preferred geographical areas. If proposals from the Ministry of Health do not fit these requirements, then other donors with more closely matched concerns would have to be approached.

The amount of aid available from donors depends on their own country's economic performance and policy on assisting those more needy than themselves. This places a limit on the total amount of aid available and therefore good negotiation skills will be vital in the competition for resources. The performance of programmes and projects that have received aid in the past is a particularly pertinent issue that needs serious consideration.

In line with these observations the Ministry of Health is working to strengthen its central planning and management capacity for donor project preparation. The steps in the process of programme or project preparation can be summarized as follows:

1 Identification and prioritization of the problem
2 Planning phase for programme or project intervention
3 Analysis of funding requirements
4 Search for sources of funds
5 Proposals for funders (government and/or foreign)
6 Donor consideration
7 Donor acceptance
8 Consultations
9 Final negotiations and signing of agreements
10 Activity programme
11 Implementation.

The persons or groups involved and the time required at each stage will vary according to whether the programme or project is for national implementation or is specific to a particular district. There may be a combination of various people involved in the preparation of programmes that are of interest to both the district and the centre.

The differences in approach are perhaps best explained by examples. For instance, a programme to support the improvement of management at Ndola Central Hospital is specific to that hospital. In such a programme, steps 1–3 should be carried out by the hospital management board, calling for advisers/consultants from Ministry of Health headquarters and from the province where necessary. Steps 4, 5 and 8 would be the specific task of the Ministry of Health, while steps 10 and 11 would be carried out jointly by the hospital management and partners from the donor body and/or the Ministry. The degree of involvement of the Ministry will depend on the ability or inability of the hospital management to produce a good quality proposal, and this in turn will have an effect on the amount of time required for preparation. Where the Ministry of Health has the local resources necessary to initiate the programme, it is expected that the preparation period will be short. For externally funded activities, the period of time required for steps 10 and 11 depends almost entirely on the donor's ability to respond.

A programme to support the control of the spread of AIDS, on the other hand, will be a national effort, with involvement from the district, province and Ministry of Health headquarters. Because the AIDS programme is a part of basic health care, there will be a lot of interest from the centre. At present, the AIDS programme is dominated by the central administration, with little or no input in terms of programme preparation at district and provincial levels. In the new scenario, the districts will submit their respective proposals and plans of action for funding, with the centre providing resources and assistance in formulation of plans. The Ministry of Health will need to take on the new role of monitoring and provision of human, financial and material resources to the districts.

A national planning workshop was held to prepare the health sector for a comprehensive plan of health investment, and a short-term action plan has been drawn up. The ministry has now embarked on a programme of establishing bilateral and multilateral agreements that are specific in terms of amounts, methods of disbursement and areas of support. This means that a lot of meetings and negotiations have to be held but in the long run it will provide an easier means of planning and management of external aid and will help the Ministry of Health ensure the successful implementation of the management information system. The initial task is to make profiles of all donors in the health sector. Voluntary agencies and technical staff have notably been left out of accounts of input in the past yet they represent an important contribution to the health sector. Methods of collecting accurate data on all technical, material and financial assistance are a priority that must receive donor support.

There is a need to ensure that details of Zambia's national health policy are made more widely available, particularly to new donors. Further, donors are to be encouraged to provide their health sector action plans to the Ministry of Health's Planning Unit for incorporation into the Ministry's calendar of activities. The Planning Unit frequently has to deal simultaneously with three or four visiting missions in the health sector, sometimes for long periods of time, leaving very little or no time for work that is pending. The Planning Unit will begin to structure visits and missions in a more manageable way and, with extra staff, the situation may improve. Where possible, donors are being asked to synchronize missions of a similar nature, such as those that focus on the same programme or project area.

Improved Ministry of Health capacity for planning and management will reduce the need for certain burdensome donor conditions, particularly those which create dependency. Donors are being encouraged to reallocate funds to support capacity-building within the Ministry of Health so that Zambian professionals may be trained to plan and manage resources effectively. Without this support, the implementation of health reforms will remain elusive.

Donors are also now being encouraged by the Ministry of Health to aim at coordinating their activities not only with the government but even with each other so that they complement each other's efforts. Many times donors want their assistance to be identified as strictly bilateral and not as a joint venture or consortium. While this may have merits in terms of easy accountability in the donor country, it puts strains on the recipient government. Coordinated sectorwide pledging should be encouraged and enhanced.

While it is important to have an efficient management information system, the Ministry of Health must move with caution in introducing a computerized system for all districts. Computerization is still a priority for the Ministry of Health. While some districts may not have a reliable electricity supply, or indeed any at all, and may at the moment be unable to provide maintenance and an ample supply of stationery, it must be part of the Ministry's future commitment to explore new technologies such as solar power and apply cost-effective systems of data storage and retrieval. Manual accounting and maintenance of epidemiological databases may prove to be not cost-effective in the long term, particularly with regard to the needs of financial monitoring. The experience of the Healthnet project, which has been implemented as a pilot project in almost all districts of three provinces, shows the merits of computerization as a future goal for a variety of purposes, not least of which is building the confidence of health workers and giving them a sense of being up to date.

Establishing quality assurance in health care

Quality health care in Zambia emphasizes the promotion and self-reliance of individuals, families and communities. Quality health care is a responsibility that is shared by the community and the care providers. It is equitable, accessible and responsive to the needs of all, especially the vulnerable groups. It provides compassionate, safe, timely, appropriate and affordable services in a suitable environment. Quality health care ensures patient satisfaction while making effective and efficient use of available health resources. It guarantees the maintenance of the professional competence of health care providers practising in acceptable working conditions. Quality health care should be monitored and assessed through reliable indicators.

A comprehensive programme to strengthen quality assurance in institutional care and primary health care has been launched through a series of district and hospital training sessions. The focus of the quality assurance activities is to:

— realize that our commitment to provide care for all translates into good care that ensures the dignity of users
— afford the opportunity to avoid harmful medicine
— maintain minimum standards
— detect variation in the quality of care
— minimize the risk of error resulting from the complexity of care.

As the concept of quality assurance is systematically applied to the practice of health care in Zambia, a continuous learning approach is being taken.

The dynamics of Zambia's reform implementation process

A systems approach to the determination of future ministerial functions has emphasized the need to reduce the size of the Ministry of Health headquarters by limiting its functions to policy guidance, reviews, monitoring, logistics support and resource mobilization during the present period of change.

When the autonomous health boards begin to exercise a more independent role, they will take over the functions of resource mobilization, personnel recruitment and small-scale logistics. This process will require time and systematic planning if the transition is to go smoothly.

Zambia's health reform efforts are typified by an emphasis on practical workable options (rather than slogans), on quality assurance in comprehensive health care, and on autonomous health authorities with the freedom to employ local innovations.

Factors that can facilitate reform include:

— favourable political climate
— dedicated leadership in the health sector
— decentralization of decision-making
— local initiatives
— well articulated policy and strategy framework
— strong donor support and coordination.

In addition, factors that may hamper reform appear to be:

— diminished purchasing power of families
— natural resistance to change
— hasty implementation without sufficient sensitization and training
— primary health care programmes heavily dependent on donors
— human resources development policy lagging behind the rest of the reform programme.

Constraints to health reforms are likely to be many and are certainly not unique to Zambia. Central policy-makers have therefore made a commitment to the three principles of leadership, accountability and partnership in initiating reforms. These principles are at the core of the policy of decentralization, building a network of smaller organizations, with less bureaucracy and regulation. The goal-oriented approach to health calls for involvement by a wide range of people in planning and decision-making relating to the coordination of services. The responsibility of the state to include more determinants of health in the provision of services places added pressure on central government. The devolution of some or all of this responsibility is therefore logical, while effectiveness will be maintained through coordination and integration of services. The transfer of responsibility for health to local level makes possible local decisions about local health needs. The health care system must be patient-centred to meet individual and community needs.

Instead of increasing bureaucratization through a centrally controlled national health service, which decreases diversity and limits social choice, we are trying to promote more diversity in policy responses to health concerns. While a pluralist approach may increase uncertainty at individual, household and health partner/provider level, it also encourages innovation and broadens the range of responses. In a society where people have differing attitudes and approaches to health, there is a need for tolerance and for mechanisms to limit conflict. Groups with differing views, such as traditional healers and private family physicians, or the opponents and proponents of abortion, should be able to interact through local structures. The decision to diversify choice and potential in health was made against the background of a socialist tradition of providing health care for a uniform society.

Our approach to health care must also stress cooperation rather than competition. The new style of health system management assumes there will be various centres of power and only a measure of cooperation between them will produce a change in the desired direction.

Past failure to integrate the mining, private and mission health approaches is evidence of the inherent competition between health care providers. The point is not to proscribe certain approaches out of existence, as has been tried. A collaborative attitude promotes a freer exchange of information, the opportunity for dialogue, the formation of shared values and ideals, and the consideration of joint solutions to shared problems if proper structures of negotiation are provided.

The sole use of present and past trends to plan for the future is particularly maladaptive in a situation of change. Health reforms must be driven by a vision of a desirable health future.

The issue of control is fundamental to planning. Being in control is basic to the responses modern societies have developed to cope with a changing environment. Mechanistic and deterministic thinking leads to such concepts as predictability and complete control.

With regard to the new health system reforms in Zambia, we have tried to plan for a situation of change and adaptation where the consequences of our actions are unpredictable, society can be influenced in the direction of a desired future but not controlled, competence is measured by the ability to learn and accept error, organizational structures are non-hierarchical, and decision-making is shared.

Increasing regulations and bureaucracy serves to rigidify our social and political institutions, reduce their ability to change and render them obsolete in a short time. Instead of regulations, we are trying to establish self-guiding mechanisms focused on values so that events may be "controlled" by influence rather than by enforcement.

When power rests with localized units, errors can be corrected more quickly. Such structures allow for greater public participation and greater local control over the means and ends in health development.

The need for continuous learning is critical to Zambia's new health vision. There is a need continuously to test new ideas and hypotheses in real life situations and learn by them, and a need constantly to revise the vision of the future that guides planning processes. Policy leaders of the health sector must be ready to learn from their mistakes.

Authoritarian and non-participative bureaucracies do not encourage creative and mutual learning. The Zambian task is to find ways of combining the technical know-how of health care staff, the pressures from people for quality health care, the structure of donor partners and the emerging collective vision in an ongoing bold experiment of health reform. This interactive and mutual learning process must emerge on the basis of mutual respect.

Respect for persons as responsible and autonomous beings is important not only for health planning but also in terms of individual health and well-being. Respect for autonomy can lead to the democratization of decision-making and can encourage citizen participation at different levels. If target populations are treated as thinking, learning and responsible people, they are likely to participate more actively in decision-making leading to a healthy society.

Although greater individual and local autonomy may appear to increase uncertainty because more variety is introduced, we in Zambia believe it is likely to lead to decisions that are more in keeping with individual and local differences. Thus cooperation, continuous learning, a future orientation, influence rather than control, and greater respect for individual and local autonomy make a sound basis for adaptation in a changing situation. Think-tanks, consultants, local workshops, meetings to build national consensus, and analytical thinking at policy leadership level are part of the broad mix of factors currently being put to work to attain Zambia's future vision for health. This is the process of social learning which we must continue to pursue, for otherwise the reform will collapse.

About the authors

Isobel Birch has worked for Oxfam since 1986. She is currently Pro-gramme Manager in Turkana, north-west Kenya, running a food distribution and pastoral development programme. She was previously a Deputy Country Representative in Zimbabwe and before that worked for several years as an administrator on Oxfam's Southern Africa desk. She has travelled extensively in Southern Africa, and is the co-author, with Robin Palmer, of *Zimbabwe: a land divided* (Oxford, Oxfam, 1992).

Paul J. Freund is a former senior research fellow of the Institute of African Studies (Community Health Research Unit), University of Zambia. He is currently Pritech Representative in Zambia promoting the use of oral rehydration therapy to combat diarrhoeal diseases. He has sat on various Ministry of Health advisory bodies and has written extensively on Zambia's health care system.

Katele Kalumba is Vice-Minister of Health in the Zambian Government. He was formerly a research fellow in the Institute of African Studies (Community Health Research Unit) and senior lecturer in the Depart-ment of Community Medicine, University of Zambia School of Medi-cine. He has authored or co-authored numerous articles in medical and health journals.

Joseph M. Kasonde was formerly Permanent Secretary and Director of Medical Services in the Ministry of Health in Zambia. He is currently with the World Health Organization in Geneva as Responsible Officer, Resources for Research, Special Programme of Research, Development and Research Training in Human Reproduction.

Kevin G. Lowther is Regional Director for Southern Africa for Africare, a Washington-based nongovernmental organization. He was Africare's representative in Zambia from 1978 to 1983 and participated in the design of the Luangwa primary health care project described in this book.

John Macdonald worked in Zambia from 1968 to 1978, latterly as coordinator of the Kaputa Joint Development Project. This project set out to coordinate the work of the churches and the government in the

116

fields of development and health. He later set up and ran a primary health care programme at Manchester University, United Kingdom. He now coordinates a primary health care programme at Bristol University, United Kingdom, and has travelled and worked extensively in the area of primary health care in Nicaragua, India, Bangladesh and several African countries. He is the author of *Primary health care: medicine in its place* (London, Earthscan, 1993) and is principal editor of the international primary health care newsletter, *Health Action*.

Margaret Malama was a health educator with the Salvation Army at Chikankata Hospital in the Mazabuka District of Zambia where she was particularly involved in community health care of AIDS patients. She later took up further studies in health education at Manchester University, United Kingdom, and is now a Programme Consultant to the Salvation Army headquarters in London.

John D. Martin was Primary Health Care Adviser in the Ministry of Health, Lusaka, Zambia from 1979 to 1982. After a period as Associate Professor in International Health at the Nordic School of Public Health in Gothenberg, Sweden, he joined the World Health Organization in Geneva where he is in the Division of Intensified Cooperation with Countires.

Mathias M. Moonde is field officer for the Lusaka Office of Africare. He served as coordinator for the first three years of the Luangwa primary health care project described in this book before joining the Africare/Zambia staff in 1985.

Vincent Musowe is Chief Health Planner in the Ministry of Health, Lusaka, Zambia.

Lumba M. Muuka-Kalumba is a freelance consultant with particular interest and experience in development economics.

Ely Nangawe is Primary Health Care Adviser in the Ministry of Health, Lusaka, Zambia.

John P. Ranken lived in Zambia from 1968 to 1970, establishing a programme of supervisory and management training at the Mindolo Ecumenical Foundation near Kitwe. From 1985 to 1991, while a senior lecturer in management at the Institute of Child Health, London, he undertook studies in Zambia concerning the work of district health managers and the role of nurse managers in support of primary health care. He helped develop proposals for an urban primary health care project in Lusaka and worked closely with the Ministry of Health's

Planning Unit to plan, implement and evaluate two three-year comprehensive management development programmes for provincial, district and local management teams.

Patrick A. Twumasi was visiting professor at the Institute of African Studies, University of Zambia, from 1983 to 1984. He is currently Professor of Sociology and Dean of the Faculty of Social Sciences, University of Ghana. He specializes in the sociology of health and social research. He has written extensively in this field, including a book currently in press, entitled *Professionalization of traditional medicine.*